CHAPTER 1
PAIN THEORY

Types of Pain

Superficial: caused by stimulation of superficial nociceptors in cutaneous tissue secondary to mechanical, thermal, or chemical injury (eg, inflammation of skin or mucous membranes).

Visceral: arises from stimulation of deeper nociceptors in the thoracic, abdominal, pelvic, or cranial cavities (eg, inflammation of an organ within the abdomen); characterized as deep, aching, cramping, or intense pressure that is diffuse and poorly localized.

Somatic: arises from muscles, joints, bones, ligaments, tendons, or fascia; characterized as sharp and severe or dull and achy, often related to changes in position; more often localized.

Pain related to metabolic need or excess: occurs as a result of insufficient blood flow to organs such as the heart, kidney, or brain (eg, atherosclerosis with plaque formation).

Neuropathic: results from damage to the peripheral or central nervous system; characterized as a burning, searing sensation that is mild to severe.

Phantom: occurs after amputation from damage to nerves; often characterized as burning with paresthesia, but sensations vary widely.

CHAPTER 2
PAIN ASSESSMENT

Assessment Strategies

Assessment is a transpersonal relationship, a sharing exchange between caregiver and client.

Assessment strategies:
- Provide privacy
- Provide client comfort
- Use open-ended questions
- Utilize therapeutic presence, projecting a caring concern

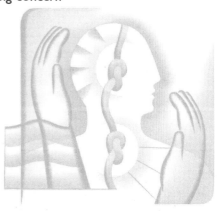

CHAPTER 1
PAIN THEORY

Interventions for Pain Based on Type

Superficial: local application of heat, cold, or pressure.

Visceral: medical or surgical interventions dependent on cause.

Somatic: medical (eg, anti-inflammatories) or surgical interventions dependent on cause.

Pain related to metabolic need or excess: rest, vasodilators, opioids, oxygen.

Neuropathic: cutaneous stimulation; opioids; antiseizure medications; relaxation, visualization, or distraction; prioritizing and pacing activities.

Phantom: teaching about cause of this pain; relaxation, visualization, stimulation of stump; have client move or massage opposite body part; anti-inflammatory medications.

This card refers to the following book:
Kazanowski MK, Laccetti MS. *Pain*. Thorofare, NJ: SLACK Incorporated; 2002.

6900 Grove Road • Thorofare, NJ 08086 • 856-848-1000
An innovative information, education and management company

CHAPTER 2
PAIN ASSESSMENT

A rapid pain assessment identifies pain in terms of:
- Type
- Severity
- Location
- Onset
- Duration
- History of previous pain

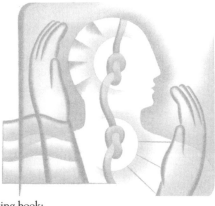

This card refers to the following book:
Kazanowski MK, Laccetti MS. *Pain*. Thorofare, NJ: SLACK Incorporated; 2002.

6900 Grove Road • Thorofare, NJ 08086 • 856-848-1000
An innovative information, education and management company

CHAPTER 3
INTERVENTIONS FOR PAIN RELIEF

Pharmacological Interventions

Nonopioid and Opioid Analgesics

For mild to moderate pain:
- Acetaminophen, aspirin, and nonsteroidal anti-inflammatory drugs
- Codeine, oxycodone, hydrocodone with or without acetaminophen or ibuprofen

For moderate to severe pain:
- Morphine, meperidine (Demerol), hydromorphone, fentanyl with or without adjuvant medications
- Local anesthetics

Medications to Treat the Cause of Pain
- Vasodilators
- Antidepressants
- Corticosteroids
- Neuroleptics
- Anticonvulsants

Physiological Interventions
- Transcutaneous stimulation
- Acupuncture
- Exercise
- Heat or cold therapy
- Reiki
- Postural changes
- Stimulation of acupressure points
- Touch: effleurage, massage, reflexology
- Therapeutic touch
- Aromatherapy

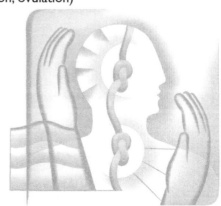

CHAPTER 4
ACUTE PAIN IN THE ADULT CLIENT

Common Causes of Acute Pain in Adults
- Trauma (eg, abrasions, contusions, burns, fractures, sprains, penetrating wounds)
- Headaches
- Cardiac disorders (eg, angina, myocardial infarction)
- Gastric disorders (eg, gastrointestinal reflux, peptic ulcer disease [PUD], inflammatory bowel disease [IBD], appendicitis)
- Dental impairments
- Pregnancy and childbirth
- Hormonal changes in females (eg, menstruation, ovulation)

Plan for Treatment of Acute Pain
- Requires client participation
- Is guided by client goals
- Is written and communicated

CHAPTER 3
INTERVENTIONS FOR PAIN RELIEF

Behavioral Interventions

- Education
- Guided imagery
- Meditation
- Hypnosis
- Relaxation
- Distraction
- Biofeedback
- Music therapy

Questions to Ask When Initiating or Altering Treatment for Pain

- Is this treatment consistent with client and family cultural or religious beliefs?
- Do the medications have maximum or ceiling doses?
- Can the client swallow this medication? If needed, can this medication be given via another route?
- If changing a route, what is the equianalgesic equivalent of the medication?
- Is the new route acceptable to the client and family?
- Will the client/family be able to administer medication via this route?
- Will cost be a factor for the client/family? Will this treatment be reimbursable for the family?

This card refers to the following book:
Kazanowski MK, Laccetti MS. *Pain.* Thorofare, NJ: SLACK Incorporated; 2002.

 SLACK INCORPORATED 6900 Grove Road • Thorofare, NJ 08086 • 856-848-1000
An innovative information, education and management company

CHAPTER 4
ACUTE PAIN IN THE ADULT CLIENT

Evaluation of Treatment Plan for Acute Pain

- Assess client acceptance, satisfaction, and adherence to the plan
- Track trends in pain episodes and treatments; assess journal or flow sheet for:
  Occurrence (time) of each pain episode
  Severity (rate using scale)
  Location of pain
  Precipitating factors
  Intervention
- Assess activities of daily living
- Assess client understanding of plan
- Verify client expectations
- Encourage consistent client feedback
- If expected outcome has not been met, reassess the client's belief in the plan and the
  availability and use of resources

This card refers to the following book:
Kazanowski MK, Laccetti MS. *Pain.* Thorofare, NJ: SLACK Incorporated; 2002.

 SLACK INCORPORATED 6900 Grove Road • Thorofare, NJ 08086 • 856-848-1000
An innovative information, education and management company

CHAPTER 5
PAIN IN THE SURGICAL CLIENT

Types of Pain Related to Surgical Procedures

Incisional: result of scalpel or trocar entry, stretching or pulling of skin tissues during surgery, irritation of surgical prep (eg, providine iodine), or tape on skin.

Somatic and visceral: result of surgical manipulation, swelling and inflammation, or fluid accumulation (eg, hematoma) around surgical area.

Neuropathic: result of surgical disruption or destruction of nerve fibers.

Other:
  Sore throat: result of intubation.
  Back and limb pain: result of positioning during surgery.

Upper back or shoulder pain: result of insufflation of abdominal cavity with gas (during abdominal or pelvic surgery).

Abdominal pain and cramping: result of decrease in peristalsis.

Calf pain: result of deep vein thrombosis—**a major complication!**

CHAPTER 6
PAIN IN THE ADULT WITH CANCER

Causes of Pain Related to Cancer
- Tumor compression of vascular structures or soft tissue
- Tumor involvement (primary or metastatic) in bone
- Infiltration of nerves by a tumor or compression of nerves by fibrosis (eg, plexopathies)
- Pathologic fracture
- Spinal cord or epidural compression
- Peripheral nerve damage secondary to neurotoxic chemotherapy (eg, vincristine, cisplatin, paclitaxel)
- Infection
- Neuralgia related to virus (eg, varicella-zoster)

Common Cancers Associated With Pain Related to Bone Metastasis
- Multiple myeloma
- Breast cancer
- Prostate cancer
- Lung cancer

Characteristics of Incisional Pain

- Cutting, searing, burning, or sharp
- More severe in locations such as the axillary area
- Increased intensity with anxiety, muscle tension

Interventions for Surgical Pain

Intraoperatively: opioids with general or regional anesthesia, or conscious sedation.

Postoperatively: NSAIDs for mild to moderate pain PRN or around the clock; opioids with NSAIDs, around the clock for first 36 hours postsurgery.

Cognitive therapies: relaxation, guided imagery, music therapy, distraction, and hypnosis.

Physical therapies: light cutaneous stimulation, deep massage, heat and cold therapies, and exercise.

This card refers to the following book:
Kazanowski MK, Laccetti MS. *Pain*. Thorofare, NJ: SLACK Incorporated; 2002.

 SLACK INCORPORATED

6900 Grove Road • Thorofare, NJ 08086 • 856-848-1000
An innovative information, education and management company

Questions to Ask When Assessing Cancer Pain

- Is this a new pain? Is the location different? Intensity? Radiation?
- What precipitated the pain (eg, trauma)?
- Is there physical evidence of trauma (eg, protruding bone or swelling in extremity related to fracture)?
- If in the periphery, are there changes in motor, sensory, or circulatory function?
- If pain is in the back, are there changes in motor, sensory, bowel, or bladder function?
- Does the client have known metastatic cancer to the bone?
- Is the client's cancer known to be associated with bone metastasis and/or spinal cord compression?

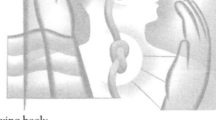

This card refers to the following book:
Kazanowski MK, Laccetti MS. *Pain*. Thorofare, NJ: SLACK Incorporated; 2002.

 SLACK INCORPORATED

6900 Grove Road • Thorofare, NJ 08086 • 856-848-1000
An innovative information, education and management company

CHAPTER 7
PAIN IN THE ADULT WITH HIV

Common Pain Syndromes Related to HIV

- Headaches
- Pharyngeal pain
- Arthralgias
- Myalgias
- Peripheral neuropathy
- Abdominal pain
- Dermatological conditions

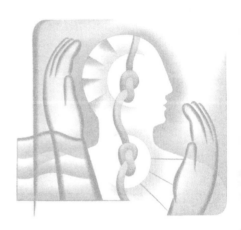

CHAPTER 8
CHRONIC BACK PAIN IN ADULTS

Causes of Acute and Chronic Low Back Pain

- Degenerative disc disease (spondylosis)
- Muscular or ligament inflammation
- Related to other disease (eg, rheumatic disorders, cancer)

Degenerative Changes that Lead to Chronic Back Pain

- Spurring with nerve root compression
- Instability
- Facet joint disease
- Disc herniation
- Spinal stenosis

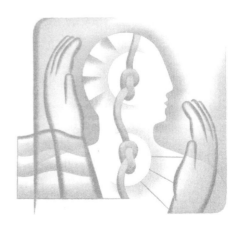

CHAPTER 7
PAIN IN THE ADULT WITH HIV

Etiologies of HIV Pain

Syndrome	Etiologies
Headaches	Infections, malignancy, antiretrovirals
Pharyngeal pain	Fungal infections, herpes simplex, Kaposi's sarcoma
Arthralgias and myalgias	Arthritis, myositis, antiretroviral medications
Myopathy (muscle weakness)	HIV infection, microsporidia, zidovudine, isoniazid (INH), ethyl alcohol (ETOH)
Peripheral neuropathy	HIV, HIV-related illnesses, medications (eg, anti-retrovirals, foscarnet, dapsone, vincristine, vinblastine)
Abdominal pain	Opportunistic bacterial, viral, or parasitic infections; hepatitis; pancreatitis; organomegaly; tumor invasion of organs; antiretroviral therapy; antibiotics
Dermatological pain	Kaposi's sarcoma, infiltration of tumors into skin or associated lymphedema

This card refers to the following book:
Kazanowski MK, Laccetti MS. *Pain*. Thorofare, NJ: SLACK Incorporated; 2002.

 SLACK INCORPORATED

6900 Grove Road • Thorofare, NJ 08086 • 856-848-1000
An innovative information, education and management company

CHAPTER 8
CHRONIC BACK PAIN IN ADULTS

Acute Pain vs.	**Chronic Low Back Pain**
Diminishes and resolves	Lacks normal checks and balances that dampen or modulate acute pain processes Occurs after tissue heals Often occurs outside area of injury

Characteristics of Myofascial Pain

- Generalized
- Radiating to hips, buttocks, groin, upper thighs
- Presence of trigger points in deep muscle

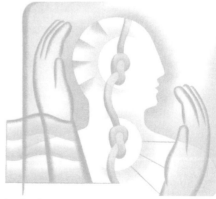

This card refers to the following book:
Kazanowski MK, Laccetti MS. *Pain*. Thorofare, NJ: SLACK Incorporated; 2002.

 SLACK INCORPORATED

6900 Grove Road • Thorofare, NJ 08086 • 856-848-1000
An innovative information, education and management company

CHAPTER 9
PAIN AND CHILDREN

Children's Reactions to Pain Based on Developmental Stages

Developmental Stage	Reaction
Neonate	Cry may not indicate pain intensity
Young Infant	Cry may not indicate pain intensity; cry will be loud and body will be rigid
Older Infant	Attempts to push away a painful stimulus; may withdraw if a history of pain; heart rate and blood pressure commonly elevated
Toddler	Loud, lusty crying and avoidance of painful stimulus; often restless, hyperactive, even when increased activity exacerbates pain
Preschool-aged child	Verbally describes location and intensity of pain
School-aged child	Verbally describes location, intensity, and type or characteristics of pain; more passive than younger children; less able to verbalize for assistance or relief than adults
Adolescent	Reluctant to communicate that they have pain; psychosocial withdrawal, decreased levels of activity; complain about issues unrelated to pain, expressing anger, suspicion, or anxiety

CHAPTER 10
PAIN AND THE ELDERLY

Factors that Increase Risk for Injury/Illness and Pain in Elders

- Decreased visual acuity
- Decreased hearing
- Changes in balance and mobility
- Loss in body mass (muscular, fatty, and subcutaneous tissue)
- High incidence of osteoarthritis
- High incidence of osteoporosis, which increases risk for fractures
- High incidence of peripheral neuropathy related to diabetes
- Increased incidence of cancer in elders
- Frequency of undergoing diagnostic procedures

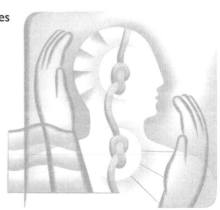

CHAPTER 9
PAIN AND CHILDREN

Pain Management Strategies for Children

Pharmacological:
- Mild to moderate pain
- NSAIDs, acetaminophen, and salicylates

Severe pain:
- Opioids
- Local anesthetics (eg, EMLA cream)
- Adjuvant medications

Physical:
- Touch, massage
- Heat and cold
- Changes in position, activity, or exercise

Behavioral:
- Soft, verbal stimulation
- Quiet environment
- Holding infant; may hold toddler if not too restrictive

With toddler—do not try to reason; give quiet, verbal commands.

With preschool-aged child—help child understand that he or she is not to blame for an illness or trauma.

With school-aged child—provide realistic choices of treatment, timing, and perhaps route of administration, but do not treat child like an adult; encourage use of familiar coping strategies.

This card refers to the following book:
Kazanowski MK, Laccetti MS. *Pain*. Thorofare, NJ: SLACK Incorporated; 2002.

 SLACK INCORPORATED

6900 Grove Road • Thorofare, NJ 08086 • 856-848-1000
An innovative information, education and management company

CHAPTER 10
PAIN AND THE ELDERLY

Factors that Increase Risks of Side Effects of Medications for Pain in Elders

- Insufficient moisture in mouth may slow or prevent dissolving of transmucosal tablets
- Fragile mucous membranes may be damaged by tablets stuck in mouth
- Difficulty in swallowing may lead to damage of mucous membranes
- Reduced stomach motility may interfere with timely absorption of oral analgesics
- Loss of subcutaneous tissue and changes in peripheral circulation may reduce transport of analgesics given subcutaneously or transdermally
- Decreased muscle mass reduces areas for storage or deposit of analgesics
- Age-related changes in liver could increase biotransformation time, resulting in longer periods of optimal or elevated serum drug levels
- Age-related changes in kidneys that affect renal clearance and excretion of analgesics, which could result in longer periods of optimal or elevated serum drug levels
- Opioid analgesics commonly cause sedation, which put immobilized elders at increased risk for side effects (eg, atelectasis, constipation, impaired skin integrity)

This card refers to the following book:
Kazanowski MK, Laccetti MS. *Pain*. Thorofare, NJ: SLACK Incorporated; 2002.

 SLACK INCORPORATED

6900 Grove Road • Thorofare, NJ 08086 • 856-848-1000
An innovative information, education and management company

CHAPTER 11
TREATMENT OF PAIN AT THE END OF LIFE

Causes of Undertreatment of Pain Near Death

- Health care providers' avoidance/denial that death is approaching
- Health care providers' avoidance/denial that pain and suffering are pertinent
- Inadequate discussion about prognosis by health care providers
- Inadequate assessment of pain and/or discomfort
- Health care providers' fear of causing respiratory depression and lethargy
- Inadequate provider knowledge about pain and symptom management at the end of life

Questions to Ask Clients When Discussing Concerns About Lingering or Serious Illness

- Do you have any pain or discomfort?
- What do you think your pain is related to?
- What helps relieve the pain?
- Are you receiving relief of your pain throughout the day? The night?
- Do you plan on having further treatment for your illness?
- Do you expect to have future hospitalizations?
- Do you have concerns about the future?

CHAPTER 12
THE VARIABLE TREATMENT OF PAIN

Factors Impacting Clients' Treatment of Pain

- Assessment of the client's pain
- Perception of the cause of the client's pain
- Expected outcome for the client's pain
- Stability of the client's pain
- Appropriateness/effectiveness of analgesics in treatment of pain
- Health care providers' knowledge related to treatment of pain
- Health care providers' concern/tolerance for pain
- Effective communication among health care agencies
- Client's access to providers who are knowledgeable and committed to relief of pain
- Agency policies related to treatment of pain

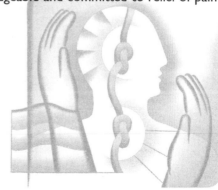

CHAPTER 11
TREATMENT OF PAIN AT THE END OF LIFE

Diseases With Prognostic Indicators for Hospice Care

- Cancer
- Renal failure
- Chronic obstructive pulmonary disease
- End-stage cardiac disease
- Amyotrophic lateral sclerosis
- Dementia
- Acquired immunodeficiency syndrome

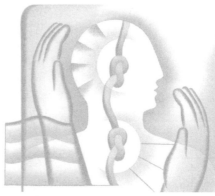

This card refers to the following book:
Kazanowski MK, Laccetti MS. *Pain*. Thorofare, NJ: SLACK Incorporated; 2002.

6900 Grove Road • Thorofare, NJ 08086 • 856-848-1000
An innovative information, education and management company

CHAPTER 12
THE VARIABLE TREATMENT OF PAIN

Essential Components of a Discharge Plan for a Client With Pain

- Comprehensive assessment of the client's pain
- Comprehensive review of recent and past treatment of pain
- Evaluation of the client's pain since most recent change in treatment
- Timing of client's pain with regard to discharge
- Written plan of care for recurrence and/or increase in pain
- Availability of effective medications for the client
- Plan of care if the client's pain does not respond to the initial discharge plan
- Plan for follow-up by a health care provider
- Verbal description of plan for treatment of pain by the client and family

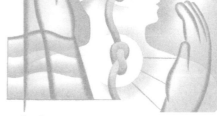

This card refers to the following book:
Kazanowski MK, Laccetti MS. *Pain*. Thorofare, NJ: SLACK Incorporated; 2002.

6900 Grove Road • Thorofare, NJ 08086 • 856-848-1000
An innovative information, education and management company

Assessment of Family Caregivers' Management of Pain Near the End of Life

- Assess family's understanding of client's prognosis
- Assess family's perception of client's comfort
- Assess family's goals regarding the client's comfort
- Assess family's beliefs about the experience of pain
- Identify family caregivers who are willing and able to administer pain medication to the client
- Assess caregivers' past experience with dying individuals
- Assess caregivers' past experience administering medication
- Assess for barriers to management of pain (eg, fear of causing injury, death; aversion to morphine; discomfort with client being sedated; inability of caregiver to administer medication via certain routes [eg, rectally])

NOTES

Nurses' Role in Instructing Family Caregivers About Medication Management of Pain

Instruct caregivers to:
- Ask client every 2 to 3 hours if he or she is having pain or discomfort
- Ask client if he or she is able to rate his or her discomfort
- Assess client every 2 to 3 hours for signs of distress (ie, grimacing, groaning, restlessness, confusion)
- Administer prescribed dose of medication at first sign of discomfort
- Evaluate client's response to the medication by asking if the pain/discomfort has been relieved; assess if any discomfort remains
- Document each episode of discomfort, medication provided, and the client's response (in terms of pain)
- If the client's pain has not been relieved to the point that the client states he or she is comfortable, contact the nurse for additional instructions
- If the client's pain or discomfort increases in frequency or intensity, or is not promptly relieved by medication, contact the nurse

This card refers to the following book:
Kazanowski MK, Laccetti MS. *Pain*. Thorofare, NJ: SLACK Incorporated; 2002.

SLACK
INCORPORATED

6900 Grove Road • Thorofare, NJ 08086 • 856-848-1000
An innovative information, education and management company

NOTES

NOTES

NOTES

NOTES

NOTES

Pain

Pain

Mary K. Kazanowski, ARNP, PhD, AOCN, CRNH
Saint Anselm College
Manchester, New Hampshire

Margaret Saul Laccetti, RN, PhD(c), AOCN
Salem State College
Salem, Massachusetts

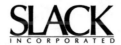

SLACK
INCORPORATED

an innovative information, education, and management company
6900 Grove Road • Thorofare, NJ 080865

Cover illustration: Thom Sevalrud
Illustrations for Figures 1-1, 1-2, 2-6, 8-1: Barbara Minnick

Kazanowski, Mary K.
　Pain / Mary K. Kazanowski, Margaret Saul Laccetti.
　　p. ; cm. -- (Nursing concepts series)
　Includes bibliographical references and index.
　ISBN 1-55642-522-8 (alk. paper)
　　1. Pain. I. Laccetti, Margaret Saul. II. Title. III. Series.
　　[DNLM: 1. Pain--nursing. WY 160.5 K23p 2002]
　RB127 .K34 2002
616'.0472--dc21   2002017652

Printed in the United States of America.

Published by:　　SLACK Incorporated
　　　　　　　　　6900 Grove Road
　　　　　　　　　Thorofare, NJ 08086 USA
　　　　　　　　　Telephone: 856-848-1000
　　　　　　　　　Fax: 856-853-5991
　　　　　　　　　www.slackbooks.com

Dedication

I dedicate this book to all the patients who have taught me so much
about the experience of pain.
Mary Kazanowski, ARNP, PhD, AOCN, CRNH

To the men in my life: my husband, Tony, and sons, Andy and BJ, for the love,
devotion, support, and occasional quiet times they so generously give me.
I carry you always in my heart.
Margaret Saul Laccetti, RN, PhD(c), AOCN

Contents

ACKNOWLEDGMENTS

I would like to acknowledge the many oncology and hospice nurses who have taught me so much about the treatment of pain. I would also like to thank my husband, Glenn, for his support in this effort.
—*Mary K. Kazanowski, ARNP, PhD, AOCN, CRNH*

I would like to recognize all of the patients and families who have trusted me to care, and who have taught me the importance of listening, hearing, hoping, and feeling in the art and science of nursing.
—*Margaret Saul Laccetti, RN, PhD(c), AOCN*

ABOUT THE AUTHORS

Mary K. Kazanowski, ARNP, PhD, AOCN, CRNH is a professor at Saint Anselm College in Manchester, NH, where she teaches medical-surgical nursing. She is also a palliative care nurse at VNA Hospice in Manchester.

Margaret Saul Laccetti, RN, PhD(c), AOCN is an associate professor of nursing at Salem State College in Salem, Mass, where she specializes in adult medicine, pathophysiology, and oncology. She received her bachelor's degree in nursing from Columbia University, New York, NY, and her master of science degree in nursing from Salem State College. She is currently in the dissertation phase of her doctor of philosophy degree in nursing at the University of Massachusetts Medical School in Worcester, where she is studying the effects of language patterns in disclosure of quality of life in end-stage breast cancer patients. She is also an advanced practice oncology nurse, whose practice includes symptom management and end-of-life issues.

INTRODUCTION

Pain is a universal phenomenon. It is experienced across all age groups, across all socioeconomic levels, and in all settings. It is one of the primary reasons why a client accesses the health care delivery system: to obtain relief from pain. Often, the health care provider is called on to intervene when the client's perceived cause of the pain requires intervention or when the pain interferes with activities of everyday living.

The pain management process is complicated. It includes assessment for the presence, type, severity, location, and possible causes of pain. Adequate and useful assessment parameters will vary widely with many types of clients. There is no one magic formula. Identification and provision of interventions to treat and prevent pain are also part of the process. An ever-expanding arsenal for pain relief is at the fingertips of health care professionals, and interventions often change depending on client goals. Continued education and an open mind to traditional as well as nontraditional approaches to pain relief provide many alternatives to use when designing a plan. Finding ways to implement the plan depends on the client's needs, beliefs, and goals; the setting; significant others; and available resources. Continuous evaluation of client outcomes and satisfaction is necessary to guide revisions to the plan and facilitate optimal pain relief. Communication among the client, family caregivers, and other health care providers is generally essential, and documentation provides evidence of the plan, its effectiveness, and revision, as well as being a tool of communication.

The 2001 Joint Commission on Accreditation of Healthcare Organizations (JCAHO)[1] has identified new standards of care regarding pain assessment and management, which will be required in any agency accredited by them. These settings include ambulatory care, behavioral health, health care networks, home care, hospitals, long-term care, long-term care pharmacies, and managed behavioral health. Basically, the standards require organizations to:[2]

- Recognize the rights of clients to appropriate assessment and management of their pain
- Identify clients with pain through an initial screening assessment
- Perform a comprehensive assessment when pain is identified
- Document assessment of the pain in such a way that will facilitate ongoing assessment and follow-up
- Educate health care providers regarding pain assessment and management
- Determine and ensure staff competency in pain assessment and management
- Address pain assessment and management in the orientation of all new staff
- Establish policies and procedures that support appropriate prescription ordering of effective pain medications
- Ensure that pain does not interfere with participation in rehabilitation
- Educate clients and families about the importance of effective pain management
- Address clients' needs for symptom management in discharge planning
- Collect data to monitor the appropriateness and effectiveness of pain management

The new JCAHO standards on pain are posted on the JCAHO website www.jcaho.org. These can be accessed by selecting "Standards Revisions for 2001" under Top Spots.

An ever-expanding arsenal of pain relief interventions are at the disposal of the health care provider. They are discovered through research, practice, and continuing education. Options are pharmacological, physiological, and behavioral. They may be traditional or nontraditional therapies. Many nontraditional therapies have roots in cultural or religious beliefs. Health care insurance providers are becoming more amenable to paying for nontraditional methods of pain control, as they are examined and determined useful through the research process. Clients are becoming more educated consumers and are often very involved in their plan for pain relief.

An important goal for the health care provider and client is not only pain relief but often pain prevention. Assessment and interventions are no longer adequate to just treat pain when it occurs, such as the common practice to prescribe pain medication to be taken as needed (PRN) when pain occurs. Rather, a new goal is to use interventions in a timely manner to prevent pain from recurring. In support of this new goal, pain management plans often include a multifaceted approach, using one or more medications in combination with a variety of other pain relief or prevention strategies.

Absolute eradication of pain is a lofty goal and is unrealistic in many situations. Optimal comfort may not equate to complete relief from pain. Clear and mutually agreed upon goals for pain relief between the health care provider and client increase the chances for success of the pain management plan. Many clients relate pain to the sense that something may be wrong or that pain means that healing or recovery is not occurring. Identification of the client's perception of pain, and client education about goals and expected outcomes increase the prospect that pain will be relieved and controlled.

Despite the existence of knowledge to identify and treat many types of pain, pain in clients remains a major problem largely because of inadequate treatment by health care professionals.

The purpose of this text is to educate health care professionals about the many barriers to quality pain management that exist within our health care system and to describe common presentations and treatment strategies for common pain syndromes. It is not our intent to include a comprehensive discussion of each type of pain and all treatment strategies. Rather, we have included selected pain experiences that we consider common problems in health care.

References

1. Joint Commission on the Accreditation of Healthcare Organizations. *Pain Standards for 2001.* Available at: http://www.jcaho.org. Accessed April 30, 2001.
2. Berry PH. Getting ready for JACHO—Just meeting the standards or really improving pain management? *Clinical Journal of Oncology Nursing.* 2001; 5(3):110-112.

Chapter 1

Pain Theory

Case Study

Mrs. R., a 39-year-old married woman, comes to the emergency department of a local community hospital complaining of severe abdominal and back pain. She is pale, diaphoretic, and nauseated. On assessment, she localizes her pain in the upper right quadrant as well as in the central portion of her back. It is unrelieved by position. Prior to coming to the hospital, she attempted to relieve the back pain through use of a heating pad. This was not successful.

> Pain, a subjective concept, is anything the individual experiencing it says it is.

Pain is a universally experienced phenomenon. It is subjective, a perception of the individual. Pain has been described as being just what the individual experiencing it says it is. Being a subjective experience, severity, duration, and meaning are determined by the individual. Pain is characterized by some objective signs and symptoms; however, assumptions cannot be made that all people will exhibit these objective signs as a part of the pain experience. Clients describe the experience as acute or chronic discomfort. In descriptive assessment, the type and severity of the pain are often characterized: agony, pulling, pressure, burning, stinging, searing, stabbing, dull aching, and so on. More than one type, sensation, or source of pain may coexist for one client at one time. It is a phenomenon that *must* be carefully assessed to plan interventions.

There are multiple and varied causes of pain. The experience can be related to trauma (major or minor), stress, surgery, illness, hormonal changes, childbirth, inflammation, and ischemia. Episodes of pain occur in the client in clinical as well as nonclinical situations. Frequently, severe pain that restricts activity or otherwise interferes with daily living is the precipitating factor for seeking out medical care. When daily living is not seriously affected, self-treatment for pain is a common choice. When self-care is not successful, medical care may become an alternative.

Acute pain usually occurs with an identifiable precipitating factor. It varies in type and severity, and may be constant or intermittent. Acuity does not refer to severity, rather it describes the time period in which the particular pain is experienced. Episodes of pain that are resolved in less than 6 months are referred to as acute. Chronic pain refers to episodes that take more than 6 months to resolve. This does not presume that the relief for acute or chronic pain cannot be successfully initiated. Rather, it indicates that the cause or precipitating factor is identified and successfully eliminated or controlled before or after a 6-month time span.

Symptoms of acute and chronic pain frequently differ on objective assessment (Figure 1-1). The client in acute pain more closely fits the stereotypical or traditional picture of pain. Activities such as grimacing, splinting, guarding, moaning, or crying are often observed, although they may not directly correlate with severity. The client with acute pain usually exhibits a change in routine level of activity, with progressively severe pain preventing successful completion of activities of daily living (ADLs). The client may become anxious or agitated with acute pain. This type of pain is seen as predictable. It can usually be controlled or eliminated; it is expected and self-limiting with the cause or precipitating factor. Physical assessment of the client in acute pain usually reveals an increase in vital signs, specifically pulse and respirations (hyperactivity of the autonomic nervous system). Blood pressure may be seen to either increase or decrease, with a decrease indicating potential for shock. The client in acute pain is frequently pale and diaphoretic.

Chronic pain is manifested quite differently. The client does not look like someone in pain by traditional standards. The chronicity of the painful experience has caused the expression of pain to differ, especially in relation to restrictions with ADLs. Chronic pain is not predictable and has no predictable end point. It is very frequently undertreated because the client is not assessed by the health care provider as being in significant pain. There is frequently no significant deviation in vital signs or other observable physiological parameters upon assessment. Fatigue and social isolation are common sequela of chronic pain. Rather than grimacing or agitation, the client in pain may exhibit slack facial features, reduced activity levels, and a flattened affect. Depression may accompany chronic pain. It is essential for the health care provider to recognize, acknowledge, and treat chronic pain as the client describes it. Treatment of chronic pain includes long-term use of prescribed interventions. With this in mind, interventions should be cost-effective or affordable, easy to understand and practice, readily available, and believable. By considering these factors for each individual client, compliance with treatment will be more commonly assured. It is also important to frequently reassess the chronic pain client.

PHYSIOLOGY OF PAIN

The sensation of pain involves both the peripheral and central nervous systems. It is primarily a warning signal to avoid injury. Response to pain is often reflexive. The central nervous system mediates other responses. Specialized nerve cells, called *nociceptors*, are sensory receptors found in skin, muscle, viscera, and connective tissue. These nerve cells respond to stimulation caused by thermal, mechanical, or chemical injury. The response is release of chemical mediators including prostaglandins. The chemical mediators cause

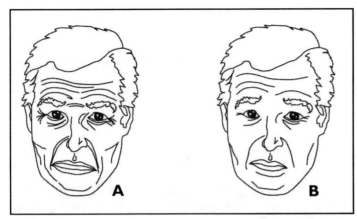

Figure 1-1. A. Acute pain denoted by obvious distress, autonomic symptoms, grimacing, and crying. B. Chronic pain denoted by not-so-obvious distress and flattened affect.

the nociceptor to "fire," carrying the pain impulse to the spinal cord. These impulses travel along afferent nerve fibers, either myelinated A-delta fibers, or unmyelinated C fibers.

The gate control theory, first proposed by scientists in 1965, argues that pain is not transmitted directly from the spinal cord to the central nervous system. Rather, a complex nerve structure in the dorsal horns of the spinal cord can inhibit transmission of the pain message to the brain. These gates operate by means of various neurotransmitters including substance P and somatostatin. Prevention of transmission to the brain also prevents the recognized sensation of pain. The injury is responded to reflexively, and the source of the unpleasant stimulus is eliminated. The stimulus only becomes pain as it is sensed consciously.

Sensory information from various areas within the body may converge at spinal neurons. This convergence is responsible for the sensation of referred pain, the pain that is perceived in a part of the body other than where the injury or stimulus has originated. By utilizing the gates in the spinal dorsal horns, a variety of methods to "close the gate" to painful stimuli are utilized to relieve or prevent pain.

TYPES OF PAIN

There is a wide variety of pain and pain sensations. The variety is a product of the multiple causes of pain as well as the unique responses to painful stimuli, especially the components of higher central nervous system responses. Pain, as discussed earlier, can be acute or chronic. Symptoms of these types are different, as are the potential interventions for control and relief. The emotional reaction of the client also changes in response to acuity or chronicity.

Superficial Pain

Superficial pain is extremely common across the life span. It is the result of stimulation of the most superficial nociceptors in cutaneous tissue, such as skin or mucous membranes. These areas are rich in afferent fibers, since one of their functions is to gather information about the world outside of the organism. Given the wealth of receptive nervous tissue in these areas, superficial pain can be experienced by the individual as quite severe or intense. Superficial or cutaneous pain may result from mechanical injury, such as scraping, abrasion, or compression (pinching the tissue). Thermal injury, including both heat and cold, is another cause of superficial pain. Finally, chemical injury causes this type of pain. It is frequently described in two distinct patterns. The first, with rapid acute onset at the time of injury, is frequently a sharp piercing or stinging sensation. The second is cutaneous pain, which arises well after the painful event and may be a deeper burning sensation that is longer lasting and more difficult to relieve. It is easily localized by the client, who can usually identify the exact location as well as the precipitating event. Potential interventions may be local—such as the application of cold, heat, or pressure—or systemic. Superficial pain is not always accompanied by obvious signs of injury. When there is obvious injury, fear, anxiety, or other intense emotions may complicate the pain and the efforts to offer relief.

Case Study Revisited

After a variety of diagnostic tests, it is determined that the source of Mrs. R.'s pain is a severely inflamed gallbladder. She is admitted to the hospital in preparation for surgical removal of her gallbladder, a cholecystectomy. Before she is transported to the surgical inpatient unit, an intravenous (IV) line is place for hydration. The nurse who is to start the IV first uses a topical anesthetic on the area to reduce the superficial pain of inserting the needle.

Mrs. R. asks the nurse what is causing her back pain. The nurse explains that this is referred pain; it is caused in a specific area of the body, here the gallbladder, but felt somewhere else. The nurse reassures Mrs. R. that referred pain to the back is very common in clients with inflamed gallbladders, and that the pain will be relieved with surgery.

Visceral Pain

Pain that arises from stimulation of deeper nociceptors may be visceral (sometimes called organ pain) or somatic (structural pain). *Visceral pain* can arise in the thoracic, abdominal, pelvic, or cranial cavities. It is diffuse, poorly localized, and frequently difficult to identify with diagnosis. Symptoms commonly associated with visceral pain are indicative of autonomic nervous system activity.

They include pallor, diaphoresis, abdominal cramping, and diarrhea. There is often a significant increase in the client's blood pressure.

> Symptoms that may accompany pain include nausea, pallor, diaphoresis, changes in pulse or blood pressure, and abdominal cramping and diarrhea.

Visceral pain may not come from the specific organ system where damage has occurred. Pressure or inflammation in surrounding tissues may cause it. One excellent example is abdominal pain accompanying intestinal disorders such as diverticulitis or colon cancer. The inside of the large intestine is poorly innervated with afferent fibers. As a matter of fact, patients with ostomies may have no sensation at the mucous membrane portion of the stoma, which is constructed from the interior of the large intestine. Rather, abdominal pain accompanying these illnesses may arise from stimulation of afferent fibers in the omentum or abdominal wall. Another source of painful stimuli is strong muscular contractions of hollow organs such as the stomach or bladder, resulting in visceral pain. Visceral pain is described as deep, aching, cramping, or intense pressure. It is this type of pain that is frequently "referred" to other areas of the body. Referred pain is a sensation that actually arises in one organ system or area of the body but is perceived by the client to be occurring in another area (Figure 1-2).

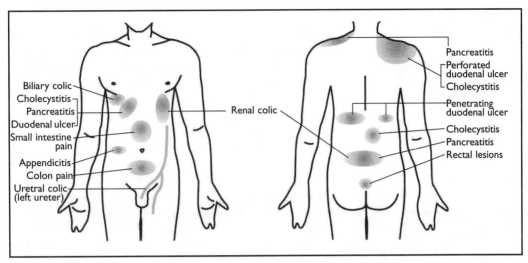

Figure 1-2. Common pathways of referred pain as they relate to an underlying abnormality.

One example of referred pain is back pain as part of the symptom set of cholecystitis. Sensation of pain at an area other than its origin may complicate timely diagnosis or delay the client's attempts to access medical care. The client experiencing back pain associated with cholecystitis may first use self-care methods such as heat, massage, and over-the-counter NSAIDs to manage the pain.

Somatic Pain

Somatic or *structural pain* is more easily localized by the client and is frequently associated with trauma or activity. It may arise in muscles, joints, bones ligaments, tendons, or fascia. The client's description of the pain may vary from sharp and severe to dull and achy. Somatic pain may be constant or intermittent, and the client often relates it to activity or positioning. Structural tissues may stimulate afferent nerve fibers because of traumatic injury such as tearing or crushing. Afferent fibers may also be stimulated by pressure, such as the result of tumor invasion, swelling, venous congestion, or chemical irritation such as in rheumatoid arthritis. Deeper somatic pain is often more poorly localized and may be experienced and reported by the client as referred pain. Clients will frequently attempt self-care measures to relieve somatic pain. This type of pain may indicate conditions that are progressive. Early intervention in these cases can prevent further injury or complications.

Pain as the Result of Metabolic Need or Metabolic Excess

Pain is often the result of metabolic need or metabolic excess in clients with vascular disease or vascular compromise. Atherosclerosis is the most common form or vascular disease. Risk factors for atherosclerosis include hypertension, hyperlipidemia, obesity, inactivity, smoking, and heredity. Clearly, many of these risk factors may be positively managed through select nursing interventions. Atherosclerosis may affect arterial or venous structures. Symptoms and treatment modalities of arterial or venous vascular disease are very different. Arterial vascular disease causes pain as the result of insufficient oxygen and nutrients in muscle or organ systems. This is *ischemic pain*. It is an excellent early warning system, since ischemic pain is experienced even when no overt damage occurs. Arterial vascular disease is central, coronary, or peripheral. Central circulation, including large vessels such as the abdominal or thoracic portions of the aorta or the carotid arteries, cause pain as the result of insufficient blood flow to organs or organ systems such as the kidneys or brain. Pain may also be the result of aneurysm formation in these vessels, compromising blood flow beyond the aneurysm. Pain also occurs as the result of direct pressure on surrounding tissues and organs when the aneurysm is quite large. Severe pain is a clinical indicator of dissection, or rupture of an aneurysm, which is a potentially life-threatening event.

Coronary artery disease accounts for a very large portion of chest pain reported to health care providers. Narrowing of the coronary arteries by atherosclerotic plaque formation, embolism, or vasoconstriction interrupts blood flow to the coronary muscle, often resulting in characteristic chest pain symptoms.

Symptoms commonly accompanying anginal or cardiac pain related to a myocardial infarction include:
- Crushing chest pain/pressure
- Pain radiating down the left arm
- Pain radiating up the left side of the neck and jaw
- Diaphoresis
- Shortness of breath
- Nausea
- Weakness

These include a sense of crushing pressure, severe pain radiating to the left arm or jaw accompanied by diaphoresis, nausea, shortness of breath, and weakness. Less common symptoms may include radiating pain to the right arm, abdominal pain, or aching sensations in the left jaw, neck, and/or arm. This pain is called *angina*. It indicates a need for oxygen to the coronary muscle but does not necessarily indicate a destructive process. When overt damage occurs to the coronary muscle, this is called a myocardial infarction (MI). Anginal pain may be relieved with rest, which decreases the oxygen deficit. It may also respond to administration of oxygen or the use of vasodilators or medications such as nitroglycerin. Opioids are not used to relieve pain during an attack of angina but may be administered to the client who has experienced an MI for management of pain as well as to reduce anxiety.

Peripheral arterial disease may be chronic or acute. The acute form occurs as the result of diminished peripheral circulation as the result of trauma, hypovolemia, or emboli. Pain is usually well localized and severe, with location depending on the arteries that are blocked. Treatment includes treating the cause, increasing oxygen transport to the area, and preventing damage below the blockage. Opioids may be used in conjunction with other treatment modalities to relieve the pain. *Heat should never be used to promote comfort when arterial compromise is suspected.* The application of superficial heat to the area results in increased metabolism. This increases the need for oxygen, exacerbates the oxygen deficit, and can result in organ or tissue damage.

Chronic peripheral arterial disease occurs as the result of progressive narrowing of the peripheral arteries and arterioles. Onset is usually subtle and insidious. The hallmark symptom is called *intermittent claudication*. This is pain that occurs with exercise and is relieved with rest. It is related to the muscle's oxygen deficit with exercise. This pain is usually reported by the client as severe, occurring in the calf. It may radiate to the thigh and buttocks. When the activity is stopped, the pain slowly recedes. Elevation of the legs does not reduce the pain; rather, keeping the legs dependent uses gravity to promote arterial blood flow. Clients with severe peripheral arterial disease report night pain, severe pain in the calf that may radiate to the thigh and buttocks, which wakes them from sleep. This pain is the result of oxygen deficit related to the reduced cardiac output during sleep and to the position of the client's legs (usually elevated in the bed). The client will report that the pain is usually resolved by dangling the legs over the side of the bed or sitting with both feet on the floor. Some clients report that this pain is so severe and frequent that they are forced to sleep in a chair, with their legs dependent. Several interventions are appropriate to promote pain relief. Clients may self-medicate with aspirin or NSAIDs. Vasodilators sometimes help. Maintaining the legs in a dependent position may prevent or relieve the pain. A supervised program of progressive exercise to the point of pain may promote formation of collateral circulation. The goal of these interventions are to promote relief and prevent tissue damage. Remember to teach clients never to use superficial heat in an attempt to relieve this pain. Many clients with severe disease elect to have surgical revascularization procedures such as arterial bypass.

> Never apply heat to an area of the body with arterial insufficiency!

Clients with peripheral narrowing of the veins from disease, compression, thrombosis, or embolization also report pain. This pain may be deep, burning, or aching. It can be constant or intermittent. It is commonly well-localized. The pain may be the result of a build-up of toxins in the surrounding tissues that are not adequately removed through venous circulation. It may be the result of inflammation or may occur because of edematous pressure on surrounding tissues. Edema occurs when valves in the peripheral veins become incompetent, allowing the column of blood to fall back with gravity, distending the veins. Valves are frequently destroyed by deposits of atherosclerotic plaque or the formation of thrombosis. Changes in pressure gradients promote the flow of fluid into the extravascular spaces. Clients with pain as the result of peripheral venous disease do not relate it to activity. Relief may be promoted through elevation or movement. Inflammatory processes that accompany thrombosis may be relieved through the use of anti-inflammatories such as NSAIDs, application of superficial heat, and elevation.

Neuropathic Pain

Neuropathic pain differs from the types of pain frequently discussed. Rather than pain that occurs as the result of information transmitted from tissue or organs via nociceptors, neuropathic pain results from damage to the peripheral or central nervous system. Stimulation of the nerves is not necessary for the client to report experiencing pain. Methods of stimulation that were not painful prior to the nerve damage may now be reported to be exquisitely painful. The reported sensations and methods for relief are very different from nociceptor pain. The pain can be mild to very severe and is frequently described as a burning, searing sensation. It is poorly localized and does not respond to conventional interventions. Neuropathic pain is commonly continuous rather than intermittent. It may be accompanied by paresthesias, sensations of heat or cold, tingling, numbness, or paralysis. As a result of the damage to the nerves, neuropathic pain often becomes a chronic symptom that can be seriously debilitating. Because the damage may not be visible and conventional relief methods useless, clients with this type of pain are sometimes considered malingerers, complainers, or noncompliant. Relief for these clients is a challenge to health care professionals. Positional changes, cutaneous, or transcutaneous stimulation may offer some relief. Use of opioids almost always fails to help. Antiseizure medications such as phenytoin (Dilantin) have been used with good effect. Nursing interventions for management of chronic pain, including relaxation, visualization, distraction, prioritizing, and pacing activities, are valuable to the client with neuropathic pain. Medical interventions may include nerve blocks and surgery.

Phantom Pain

One specific form of neuropathic pain occurs after an amputation. This is called *phantom pain*. It is pain experienced by the client in the portion of the body that has been amputated. It is not a function of the client's imagination. Phantom pain arises from damage to nerve fibers at the stump. The type of pain varies widely but is often accompanied by sensations similar to other types of neuropathic pain, including burning sensations and paresthesias. The client may also report sensations that feel like the missing limb is in an uncomfortable or cramped position. Nursing interventions for phantom pain include teaching about this very real phenomenon. Fear, anxiety, misunderstanding and denial, or reluctance to report the pain inhibit attempts at providing relief. Relaxation, visualization, and having the client imagine moving the missing area into a more comfortable position are sometimes helpful. Stimulation at the stump may also relieve some of the phantom sensation. Another alternative to promote relief includes having the client move or massage the opposite body part (the right foot if the left foot is missing). Anti-inflammatory medications are sometimes helpful in the acute stages following the amputation. Opioids are limited in their effect. Other interventions for neuropathic pain are helpful in relieving phantom pain.

VARIABLES AFFECTING PAIN

A variety of variables may affect the pain experienced by the client. They can include mood, anxiety, fear, stress, powerlessness, anger, reluctance to discuss pain, shame, sleeplessness, fatigue, and culture. These variables affect the expression of pain, as well as its severity and meaning in the client's life. For many of these variables, a circuitous pattern may be established, with pain enhancing the variable while the variable exacerbates the pain.

Clients in pain frequently suffer from depression. This may range from a simple case of the blues to a long-term clinical depression warranting medical intervention. The depression may be related to the experience of pain itself or may revolve around issues such as diagnosis, immobility, change in role, or body image changes. Depression may also be a variable that exists independent of the pain experience, yet is an exacerbating factor. The client who is depressed may have increased experience of pain. This client may have difficulty in reporting pain, seeking relief, or compliance with a pain relief regimen. Although depression is often associated with chronic pain, it may be a factor for the client in acute pain as well. Symptoms of depression include flattened affect, reported feelings of sadness, decreased pleasure or interest, changes in appetite and sex drive, and sleep disturbances. Assessing for and offering interventions for depression will result in a greater potential for optimal pain relief.

Fear, anxiety, and increased stress may exacerbate pain as well as introduce barriers to pain relief. *Fear* is a sense of discomfort with a defined or specific stressor. It may be fear of tests, treatments or procedures, a diagnosis, or an outcome. Clients fear death, pain, and situations that are potentially painful. Many other specific items or ideas may be feared.

Fear can impede the client's ability or willingness to seek out diagnosis or treatment for pain. The client who fears needles will certainly be reluctant to use a pain relief option that involves intramuscular or subcutaneous injections. Not all fears are rational, obvious, or easily understood by the health care provider. Through careful and sensitive assessment, stressors that are feared may be identified. Once identified, they can be addressed and managed to enhance client comfort.

> Many patients are fearful of injections, making this a difficult route to administer pain medication. Several strategies can be used to deal with this fear. First, consider a different route for administration of the medication. Alternatives include oral, rectal, transdermal, topical, or transbuccal (across the mucous membranes). If another route is not an alternative, use of relaxation or distraction may help. Try to allow the client to have some sense of control, perhaps choosing timing or site of the injection. Finally, intramuscular injections are much more painful when given into a tensed muscle. Assist the client into a comfortable position that allows for relaxation of the muscle where the injection will be administered.

Anxiety is a sense of uneasiness or discomfort with no concrete causative factor or specific stressor. Given the more vague, global nature of anxiety, it is sometimes more difficult to manage. Anxiety, like fear, may present significant barriers to diagnosis and treatment. In addition, physiological changes may accompany anxiety, which cause or exacerbate pain. Increased muscular tension and metabolism are frequently seen symptoms of anxiety. Increases in muscular tension can cause pain, such as the all too common tension-related headache. Muscular tension can also exacerbate existing pain syndromes. It can also cause diagnostic- or treatment-related procedures to be much more difficult and painful. A calm, professional attitude on the part of the caregiver is essential in helping the client to deal with anxiety. Privacy, a comfortable environment, minimal waiting time, and reduced cues to anxiety will also help. Relaxation techniques, guided imagery, music therapy, breathing exercises, and distraction are several other strategies for helping the client to reduce anxiety. Finally, adequate, clear information and direct instruction are useful in offering the anxious client intervention for pain. When someone is fearful or anxious, it is often difficult for him or her to listen,

> Some ways to decrease anxiety include progressive relaxation, guided imagery techniques, distraction, listening to music, controlled breathing exercises, client teaching, information sharing, and therapeutic presence.

attend to a situation, and retain information. Concentration is a major effort. Speak slowly, clearly, and repeat important information or instructions. Written, audiotaped, or videotaped information may be other methods of sharing information. Stress that is unrelated to the client's pain or medical condition can frequently lend other anxieties or fears. Pain does not occur independent of the rest of the client's life. It is important to attempt to assess for other stressors to prevent their interference with pain management.

It is very important to assess clients' learning styles when providing client teaching. If providing verbal or auditory information, assess for language and hearing. Consider the client's ability to read and visual acuity when providing written information. Use return demonstration and open-ended questions to attempt to assess understanding and retention of information shared. Repeat important points or concepts. Remain open and available for questions. Remember, anxiety and pain are significant barriers to learning.

Powerlessness is a sense that no action taken on the part of the individual will result in change. Powerlessness may be related to disease, diagnosis, or prognosis. A change in roles may force the client to relinquish decision-making, enhancing a sense of powerlessness. Situational powerlessness may occur in interactions between the client and health care providers when information is withheld or control is usurped by the health care team. It can also be related to lack of knowledge, physical disabilities, isolation, and chronicity of pain. The client who perceives himself to be powerless in pain relief presents a challenge similar to the client suffering from depression.

Anger is a powerful destructive force, using large amounts of energy to sustain. It is exhausting and a barrier to communication and pain relief. The client may be angry at something that is related to his or her illness or pain; however, the anger may be completely unrelated. Assisting the client to resolve anger will help to reduce barriers to pain relief.

Sleep disturbances and fatigue are often associated with pain. *Fatigue* is feeling tired unrelated to sleep or energy expended. It is not relieved by rest and can be severely debilitating. It is associated with multiple disease states including anemia, cancer, and depression. Fatigue is frequently related to chronic pain. It can be implicated in reducing the client's tolerance for pain as well as a barrier to seeking out intervention or being proactive in pain management. Pain is one primary reason for sleep disturbances. Certain pain medications, including opioids, may interfere with REM (rapid eye movement) stage sleep, reducing the benefits of the time spent sleeping. Sleep deprivation can affect the client's ability to deal with pain in similar ways to fatigue. It can also make it difficult for the client to concentrate and communicate effectively. Sleep deprivation can be resolved by identifying and correcting the causes.

The client's cultural background may affect the way pain is experienced, manifested, reported, or described. It may determine the meaning of the pain in the client's life. Culture also determines the appropriateness of certain interventions. Finally, the culture of the client or caregiver can introduce certain biases into the pain intervention process. Culture may dictate how a client manifests his or her pain. It may also result in differences in manifestation between men and women. In some cultures, stoicism in the face of pain is required, inhibiting assessment and preventing intervention. In other cultures, especially in certain situations, pain is openly and verbally expressed. At times, these expressions may appear to the health care provider to be out of proportion with the perceived severity of the pain. It is important for the nurse not to allow biases or cultural differences to interfere with assessment or intervention.

The culture of the client or the caregiver can be a source of bias about pain, its manifestations, and pain relief. It is important to never make unsupported assumptions on the basis of culture or gender alone. To do this may hinder attempts to assess or relieve pain.

Case Study Resolved

Within 3 hours of her admission to the hospital, Mrs. R. has her gallbladder removed. Her pain is well-managed through use of a PCA (patient-controlled analgesia) pump, on which the nurse provided instruction for both before and after surgery. The PCA pump is discontinued 24 hours after surgery in preparation for Mrs. R.'s discharge to home. She complains of some lower abdominal pain, which is crampy in nature. The nurse explains this may be gas pain, which may be relieved through increasing physical activity. Mrs. R. ambulates several times along the hallway and later reports good relief from the pain.

BIBLIOGRAPHY

Acute Pain Management Guideline Panel. *Acute Pain Management: Operative or Medical Procedures and Trauma. AHCPR Pub No. 92-0032.* Rockville, Md: Agency for Health Care Policy and Research, Public Health Service, US Department of Health and Human Services; 1992.

Carrieri-Kohlman V, Lindsey AL, West CM. *Pathophysiological Phenomena in Nursing.* Philadelphia, Pa: WB Saunders Co; 1993.

Karch AM. *2002 Lippincott's Nursing Drug Guide.* Philadelphia, Pa: Lippincott; 2001.

MULTIPLE-CHOICE QUESTIONS

1. Pain can be best described as:
   A. An objective phenomenon, primarily characterized by observable signs and symptoms
   B. A symptom consistently seen with trauma or disease
   C. A subjective phenomenon, perceived by the individual, and characterized by what the individual says it is
   D. A symptom that has no particular relation to the illness or trauma

2. When pain is severe and restricts or limits activities of daily living, the client will commonly:
   A. Self-medicate
   B. Seek out medical intervention
   C. Limit all social interactions
   D. Identify the precipitating factors before seeking relief

3. The client experiencing chronic pain:
   A. Exhibits crying, grimacing, and other classic symptoms
   B. Severely limits activities
   C. Is pale and diaphoretic
   D. May appear to have no observable symptoms

4. Common signs and symptoms associated with acute pain include:
   A. Increase in pulse and respiration, pallor, and either increase or decrease in blood pressure
   B. Ruddy complexion, bradycardia, and shortness of breath
   C. Decrease in pulse, respirations, and blood pressure
   D. Syncope and diaphoresis

5. The sensation of pain involves:
   A. The peripheral nervous system
   B. Both the peripheral and central nervous systems
   C. The autonomic nervous system
   D. The central nervous system

6. The gate control theory argues that:
   A. All pain sensations must be passed through a series of gates to be perceived and acted upon
   B. Gates that are active in transmitting messages of pain operate through the use of prostaglandins
   C. A complex structure in the dorsal horns of the spinal cord can inhibit the transmission of pain; the gate is then closed
   D. Only reflexive reactions occur in response to pain

7. One common example of pain that occurs as the result of metabolic need or excess is:

    A. Pain as the result of myocardial infarction

    B. Migraine headache

    C. Trauma-induced pain

    D. Labor

8. Intermittent claudication, the hallmark symptom of chronic peripheral arterial disease, is characterized by:

    A. Severe, unrelenting chest pain at night

    B. Pain in the legs that occurs with exercise and is relieved by rest

    C. Pain in the calf that occurs when legs are raised and is relieved by moving to a leg-dependent position

    D. Numbness, pain, and blanching of the fingers and toes

9. All of the following are characteristics of neuropathic pain except:

    A. Neuropathic pain is successfully relieved through the use of morphine

    B. Neuroleptic medications may be used in the treatment of neuropathic pain

    C. Neuroleptic pain is more commonly persistent, rather than intermittent

    D. A particular type of neuropathic pain is phantom pain

10. A client's cultural background:

    A. Never affects the way pain is perceived or expressed

    B. Always presents a significant barrier to pain management

    C. May determine the appropriateness or acceptability of an intervention

    D. Is not useful in determining a plan of care for the client in pain

MULTIPLE-CHOICE ANSWERS

1. C. Pain is subjective, may have no observable manifestations, and should be recognized as being whatever the individual experiencing it says it is.
2. B. When pain limits normal activities, the client will seek medical intervention. If pain does not restrict activities or daily living, self-medication is usually attempted.
3. D. The client in chronic pain may have no observable traditional signs and symptoms of pain, yet may still be experiencing severe pain that needs intervention. It is more difficult for the nurse to assess.
4. A. Increase in pulse and respiration, pallor, and either increase or decrease in blood pressure are indicative of hyperactivity of the autonomic nervous system associated with acute pain.
5. B. Both the peripheral and central nervous systems are used in sensing pain.
6. C. Pain is not transmitted directly from the peripheral to the central nervous system, but through a gate or complex nervous structure in the dorsal horn of the spinal cord through various neurotransmitters including substance P and somatostatin.
7. A. The pain resulting from myocardial infarction is the product of oxygen deficit.
8. B. Pain that occurs with exercise and is relieved by rest is caused by oxygen deficit and lactic acid build-up in the calf muscles, relieved by rest and elevation of the legs.
9. A. Opioids are rarely useful in the treatment of neuropathic pain.
10. C. A client's cultural background may determine if an intervention or the health care professional who offers the intervention is appropriate, acceptable, or useful for that particular client.

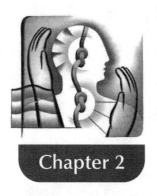

Chapter 2

Pain Assessment

Case Study

Mr. A., a 68-year-old retired engineer, comes to the senior center health clinic with the complaint of leg pain. His wife accompanies him on this visit. He is able to ambulate independently, walking without assistance into the exam room. According to the client, the pain is in both legs and happens when he walks and at night during sleep.

Prior to designing or implementing an intervention for a client's symptom or problem, the nurse must be able to assess the problem. A comprehensive pain assessment is essential to identifying interventions appropriate for each specific client and each specific episode of pain. Assessing for pain includes collecting both subjective and objective data. Initial, rapid assessment of the client in pain should include identification of the type, severity (or intensity), onset, duration, location, and previous history of the pain. Both effective and noneffective self-care strategies should also be elicited. The pain experience should be described in the client's words. Some clients may avoid using the word *pain* and actually deny pain as a problem, preferring to use a word such as *discomfort*. Acknowledgement of the client's personal description is essential to establishing effective communication, and this description is adhered to in subsequent assessments.

Additional data in a comprehensive pain assessment includes identification of physiological signs and symptoms of pain, vital signs, a medical history, and assessment of psychosocial and cultural factors (Table 2-1). The American Pain Society has challenged all health care systems to make pain the fifth vital sign. Making pain a vital sign would ensure that pain is monitored on a regular basis and would ideally signal a need for further assessment and treatment.

Table 2-1
Rapid Pain Assessment A rapid pain assessment includes: • Type • Severity • Location • Onset • Duration • History of previous pain

A health care professional's personal or cultural biases about pain and pain relief can negatively impact a pain assessment. The biases may prevent a nurse from viewing the client's expression of the pain as valid or meriting intervention.

Incomplete data collection, especially when related to health care provider biases or assumptions about pain, can lead to failure to offer useful interventions or cause further harm to the client. The client's pain sometimes impedes comprehensive assessment. Full assessment can be time-consuming; a variety of assessment and documentation strategies are useful in streamlining the task of assessing the client in pain.

ASSESSMENT STRATEGIES

Assessment is a transpersonal relationship, a sharing exchange between caregiver and client. The client trades knowledge or information for high-quality nursing care. The care-

Assessment is an essential step in providing adequate pain relief. It is conducted initially and regularly throughout the client's treatment or illness trajectory.

giver would be unable to design a plan of care that is specific to the needs of the client without assessment information. In using the assessment to identify problems and past interventions, the health care professional provides the structure for the exchange. Several strategies are useful in structuring and streamlining the assessment process.

Privacy is fundamental to the assessment process. Much of the information revealed during assessment is of a personal nature, not easily shared under uncomfortable circumstances. A private, comfortable area should be available to conduct assessment activities. In addition to protecting the client and maintaining confidentiality from strangers, it is also a matter of health provider judgment whether or not to exclude the significant other from all or part of the assessment process. For many clients, the presence of a spouse or parent is a comfort; but in other instances, the nature of the information shared is confidential. Clients may choose to protect family from knowledge of the severity of the pain.

Methods of pain relief may also be confidential. Without privacy, the facts of the client's pain may not be fully disclosed. In another circumstance, the significant other may attempt to answer all assessment questions for the client. In this situation, only the significant other's perception of the client's pain is assessed. Pain is a subjective experience. Assessment should primarily include the client's perspective. Use of the significant other's input in addition to thorough client assessment may be useful.

Imaginative strategies must sometimes be used to convince a family member to leave the room during an assessment. Sending him or her on an important errand, such as retrieving old medical records or x-rays from another location, is one possibility. Giving him or her permission to indulge is another option ("Go get some coffee and relax for a while." "Have you eaten dinner yet?" "You must be hungry.") The client may be reluctant to ask a family member to leave. You might also ask a family member to step outside while you perform some sort of procedure while continuing your assessment. Most family members are comfortable with leaving the client if a medical or nursing task must be done.

When a client is uncomfortable, assessment may be hindered. The environment where an assessment is conducted should be clean, well lit, and relatively free of distractions. A chair may be more comfortable than an exam table for some clients. The temperature of the area should be warm enough for the client who is only partially clothed or a blanket should be provided. Attempts should be made to minimize interruptions. When the nurse is forced to respond to multiple requests or tasks during the assessment, important information may be missed. It is also important to maintain control of the interview, restricting the discussion primarily to the area of desired information. Many clients, especially the elderly or isolated clients, regard the assessment interview as an opportunity to visit or socialize. Assessment is essential to providing client care. Through minimizing distractions, interruptions, and extraneous information, the process will take less time and be more productive.

As in many client interactions, it is important to remember to ask open-ended questions during the pain assessment, allowing the client freedom to respond. This practice will enhance information shared and prevent caregiver biases from obscuring client data. Incorporating a framework into the assessment process assists in obtaining data and identifying missing elements.

Examples of open-ended questions:
- Tell me about your pain.
- Describe how you are feeling.
- What does it feel like?
- Tell me how this began.
- What other experiences have you had with pain?

Two examples of assessment framework commonly used by nurses include head-to-toe assessment and functional health patterns. Choosing a framework should reflect the nurse's personal comfort and knowledge, as well as the structure of documentation required.

While conducting a pain assessment, the provider utilizes therapeutic presence, projecting an air of caring concern. Clients will not share information with a professional whom they perceive to be uninterested or distracted. Body language is one component of this presence. During the interview, the provider should appear receptive with professional dress and posture, and hands still and visible. The provider should sit at the same level as the client, avoiding a position of authority over the client. When culturally appropriate, the provider should also maintain eye contact. One should speak in a clear, calm tone, using language and terms easily understood by the client and verifying the client's understanding of the questions asked.

BARRIERS TO ASSESSMENT

Just as an inadequate assessment is a barrier to pain management, there are many barriers to the assessment process. Pain is one of the primary barriers. The client suffering from pain has a shortened attention span and may not communicate clearly. The pain inhibits the client from comprehending other stimuli. In such an instance, the pain becomes an obstacle to efforts for relief.

The mental status of the client can be another barrier, which may or may not be pain-mediated. Anxiety, which often accompanies pain, reduces comprehension, memory, and the ability to communicate. A client in pain may experience significant anxiety as a byproduct or related to hospitalization, treatment, diagnostic procedures, role difficulties, or a variety of factors totally unrelated to his or her state of health. Acknowledging and addressing the state of anxiety and possible causes may be necessary prior to a pain assessment. If this is not possible, several steps can be taken to accommodate the anxious state. The provider should make an effort to speak slowly and clearly, frequently validating the client's understanding of questions and client responses. A quiet, nonthreatening environment should be maintained, and activities should be varied to accommodate the client's shortened attention span. For example, questions can be interjected while performing parts of the physical assessment. Severe anxiety may necessitate using an alternate history source, such as the client's family member or medical record.

Confusion is another problem that may interfere with assessment activities. It may be the result of a physiological condition such as hypoxia, blood loss, low blood pressure, hypoglycemia, electrolyte imbalances, medication ingestion, psychological disorders, or central nervous system disease. Other factors implicated in confusion include changes in diet and nutritional status, changes in environment and routine, trauma, and age. The elderly and very young are more apt to become confused when removed from a familiar environment, routine, and caregivers. Identifying the related factors to confusion and attempting correction when possible (such as administration of oxygen in a hypoxemic client) may allow for a more comprehensive pain assessment.

The client's physical condition, in addition to pain, may impede conducting a pain assessment. The client may be severely hard of hearing, comatose, or unable to communicate. Careful assessment for any signs of discomfort, such as grimacing at rest or with movement, is important. Time is a common barrier to comprehensive assessment, both because the client may not be physically present or available for prolonged periods and because of multiple demands placed on the provider's time. Organizational skills and realistic ordering of priorities may help resolve the problem of time constraints.

Limited time should not impede an adequate assessment. Pain assessment is not a luxury: it is a requirement for provision of adequate care.

Language and culture are two other potential barriers to pain assessment. Culture dictates the value and meaning of the pain experience, as well as the conditions around disclosure. In some oriental cultures, pain is experienced stoically—neither complained about nor even described. In other cultures, pain is expected and, in

> Culture dictates the value, meaning, and demonstration of pain. It may also impede communication about pain either from the client's cultural perspective or the heath care professional's cultural biases.

some instances, loudly vocalized. One example of this is childbirth during which in certain cultures the mother loudly proclaims her discomfort. It is part of the ritual of giving birth. Language, as a cultural barrier to assessment, is problematic when an appropriate interpreter is unavailable. It is important to note that many clients who speak English as a second language are much better able to communicate in their primary language during periods of intense stress or discomfort. Family members should not be used as interpreters, if at all possible, to maintain client confidentiality and to ensure factual information. Language may also inhibit the assessment process when the client or health care provider does not understand the other's use of medical jargon, street vernacular, or slang.

The environment in which an assessment is conducted can provide multiple barriers to the process. Noise, frequent interruptions, a sense of lack of privacy, discomfort, and depersonalization can be part of the health care facility's environment. Depersonalization occurs when the client perceives that he or she is not valued or respected as a person and that what he or she is saying is not being listened to or used in planning his or her care. This may be a direct result of fear or distrust of the health care system or providers, or may be related to the attitude or actions of the health care provider. Minimizing the importance of a client's input, treating him or her like a child, or reducing his or her ability or opportunity to make realistic decisions concerning his care also contributes to a sense of depersonalization.

The immersion of a client in the sick role may also be responsible for depersonalization. The role of an ill individual often includes relinquishment of activities and responsibilities. However, it should also include efforts to return to a state of good health with a goal of participation in activities of daily living.

Hopelessness or powerlessness can have a major impact on the client's participation in the assessment process. If the client perceives that nothing can be done to relieve his or her pain or that he or she, personally, is unable to participate in productive activities to provide pain relief, participation in the pain assessment will be minimal. Listening to the client, assessing for flattened affect, reluctance to participate, or a history of conflict with health care providers will indicate clues to hopelessness or powerlessness.

Finally, lack of access to a competent historian may inhibit pain assessment. There should be documentation as to who is providing the history. If the source is not the client, the perception of the pain experience is objective, not subjective.

Case Study Revisited

The nurse begins Mr. A.'s assessment with a pain history. She asks him to describe his pain, to which he responds: "It is a throbbing, aching pain in both legs, mainly my calf area, but sometimes it feels like it goes up to my thighs." His wife adds: "It's his whole leg that hurts!" The nurse then asks how long the client has had the pain and if it is constant or intermittent. Mrs. A. replies: "It hurts him all the time, he doesn't even sleep at night. Stop asking all these questions. We just want to see the doctor."

Realizing that the A.'s don't understand the process of assessment, the nurse explains quietly. She then arranges for Mrs. A. to leave the room to provide insurance information. Using this short interval of privacy, she encourages Mr. A. with open-ended questions to describe the duration and quality of his pain. She shows him a linear numeric pain scale and he describes the severity of his pain as "6 to 8 when it occurs"; however, he is pain-free at this particular time. He explains that the pain interferes with his sleep, waking him frequently at night. The pain also interferes with his favorite leisure activity, playing golf. The pain usually occurs when he walks, even slowly, for more than 5 minutes.

OBTAINING A PAIN HISTORY

The initial step in a comprehensive pain history is to interview the client, collecting a subjective history of the pain. Using the strategies discussed previously, the nurse asks open-ended questions about the type, location, severity, and nature of the pain. Listen carefully to the descriptors offered by the client. His description of the pain may indicate the source or type of pain. One excellent example is the *burning, hot feeling* described by the client suffering from herpetic shingles. The pain results from the inflammation of the nerve along which the herpes lesion is growing. Nerve pain, or neuroleptic pain, is commonly described using words like *hot, burning, searing,* or *scalding*. The competent historian responds to these clues when designing interventions. Neuroleptic pain does not commonly respond to narcotics, making them a poor choice for relief with this type of pain.

Location of the pain should be as specific as the client can describe. Avoid broad descriptive terms like "stomach ache." Determine where the pain originates and if it radiates to other areas of the body. If pain is present in more than one area of the body, does the client relate the pains, or feel they are separate occurrences? Investigate what exacerbates or diminishes the pain. Identify activities that provide relief, such as change in position, eating, emptying the bladder. Identify measures the client has tried for pain relief and their effect.

Determine how long the client has been in pain. Assess if it is a recent occurrence or the intensification of a chronic condition. While assessing duration, ask about the consistency of the pain. Find out if it is constant and unremitting, or if it is intermittent in nature. If the pain is intermittent, ask if there is a cyclic quality, or if the pain recurs with some identified stimulus. Does the pain occur at certain times of the day or night? Does it cause the client to awake from sleep?

Intensity or severity of pain is assessed using a pain scale, allowing for rating of the pain. A variety of imaginative scales are available for use, and choice of scale is determined by the client's ability to communicate the intensity of the pain most accurately. A linear analogue or visual analogue (Figure 2-1) is considered the easiest for adults. This scale utilizes a line with qualifiers at one end, such as 0 (no pain), and 10 at the opposite end, indicating the worst pain one could ever imagine. Numeric scales will often utilize numbers from 0 to 10 at regular intervals (Figure 2-2). The client indicates how severe his or her pain is along the linear scale. The Acute Pain Management Panel[1] recommends standardizing linear and numerical scales along a 10 cm line. Standardized scales provide the opportunity for enhanced communication about the pain.

A descriptive scaling of pain is an alternative for assisting a client in his or her rating of the pain. Words are placed in order of severity (such as no pain, mild discomfort,

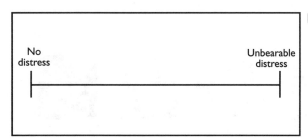

Figure 2-1. Visual analog scale (VAS).

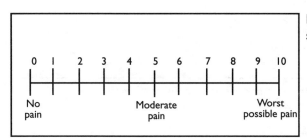

Figure 2-2. 0 to 10 numerical pain intensity scale.

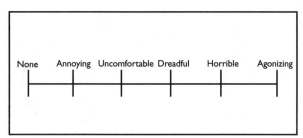

Figure 2-3. Simple descriptive pain distress scale.

painful, terribly painful, and unbearable pain). The provider reads the words to the client and asks him or her to choose the descriptor that best describes the severity of the pain. Numbers correspond with each descriptor, with 0 indicating no pain, 1 indicating mild pain, etc; the the higher the number, the more severe the pain (Figure 2-3).

Standard scales for description of pain severity enhance communication, validate successive interventions, and provide more reliable evaluation of relief methods. Standard scales help us all to speak the same language about the pain. The use of these scales also aids in comparing pain from one instance to another or even one individual to another. This gives us a basis for research-based practice.

A variety of other visual pain scales have been developed for use in assessment. Some include the use of color, either in discrete blocks or shading. These may be combined with descriptive words or numeric ranking (Figure 2-4). It is important to note that color may be interpreted differently by different cultures. Color may also be more expensive to duplicate when copying the scale for the use of other heath professionals. Line drawings or cartoons of simple facial expressions ranging from happy through grimacing are useful with children and nonverbal client populations (Figure 2-5).

Assess for symptoms that accompany the pain. These may include dizziness, photosensitivity, a sensation of light-headedness or feeling faint, nausea, diaphoresis, flushing or pallor, incontinence, weakness, loss of balance, redness, swelling, or warmth. Also

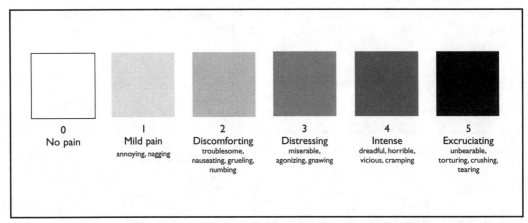

Figure 2-4. Pain assessment ruler (note: ruler is commonly in color. 0 = white; 1 = light blue; 2 = yellow; 3 = light orange; 4 = dark orange; 5 = red).

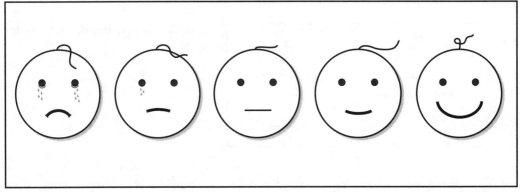

Figure 2-5. Scale to assess pain in children (adapted with permission from Ada G. Rogers, RN [retired], Memorial Sloan-Kettering Cancer Center, New York, NY).

assess for comorbidities: health problems that may change perception of pain or may impact the choice of interventions.

In assessing the nature of the pain, ask what impact it has on the client in terms of affecting mood, habits, and ability to participate in activities of daily living. Ask if the pain impacts sleep or rest, eating, mobility, or sexuality. Has the pain affected family dynamics or function in the

> Frequently, clients do not seek medical care until their symptoms interfere with everyday life or are resistant to attempts at self-care.

workplace? Assess what the client suspects is the cause. Finally, ask the client to describe his or her history of pain: has he or she ever had pain like this before? What relieved the pain? What are his or her other experiences with pain and pain relief, especially medications? Identify allergies or sensitivities to medications and current use of prescribed and unprescribed medications.

At the conclusion of a thorough pain history, the health care provider verifies information obtained with the client to avoid misunderstandings or incomplete data.

Case Study Revisited

Mr. A. describes how he has been managing his pain. He says at night, the pain goes away when he dangles his legs off the bed and sits with his feet on the floor. Some nights it comes back again four or five times when he is asleep. For the past two nights, he has slept in a chair with his legs down. Both he and his wife find this very distressing.

When questioned about the pain that occurs with exercise, he states: "It goes away when I rest." The nurse determines that elevating his legs does not provide relief. The pain first occurred about 7 months ago, just with exercise. The pain at night began to occur 6 or 7 weeks ago. Mr. A. seeks treatment now because he feels that his life has been seriously affected. He denies using any medications for the pain. "I tried taking aspirin, but it didn't help." He is allergic to clarithromycin (Biaxin) but no other medications. "I've always been a healthy guy," he tells the nurse. "I have never had pain like this in my life. I want it to go away so I can enjoy my life, or at least get a good night's sleep."

PHYSICAL ASSESSMENT

The physical assessment for pain involves identification of objective signs of pain. Although pain is primarily subjective, objective manifestations can be of value, especially when evaluating interventions for relief. It is not the goal of the pain assessment to diagnose the cause of pain. A rapid head-to-toe assessment can identify contributing factors as well as barriers to assessment. Vital signs may indicate a painful state, usually with an increase in heart rate, respirations, and an elevation in blood pressure. However, in some clients, blood pressure may decrease with severe pain. State of consciousness and affect may vary with severe pain. Agitation is often associated with acute pain, while a flattened affect of withdrawal may be associated with chronic pain. Physical assessment of the painful area includes evaluation for redness, swelling, heat or cold, masses, and a functional assessment. Functional assessment includes sensation and movement of an affected extremity, bowel sounds in a painful abdomen, or heart and breath sounds in the case of chest pain. Physical assessment progresses from inspection through auscultation, then percussion (when these are indicated) to palpation. Percussion and palpation may exacerbate the client's pain. The client is asked to demonstrate positions or movements that increase or relieve the pain. Throughout the physical assessment, privacy and comfort are provided.

A physical examination is done in addition to a pain history, not as a replacement for the history. A client's self-reported history reveals subjective symptoms. A physical exam identifies objective signs. Pain is a subjective phenomenon.

The order of techniques in a physical assessment is:
- Visual inspection
- Auscultation
- Percussion
- Palpation

Case Study Revisited

On physical assessment, Mr. A. is found to have vital signs within normal limits, except for a mildly elevated blood pressure of 140/86. According to his medical record, this is his normal baseline pressure. Both legs are thin, pale, and almost hairless from the knee down. His calf muscles appear wasted, and there is no excess adipose tissue. His feet are cool, with fair capillary refill. There are no areas of redness, swelling, or heat. No ankle edema is noted. He reports feeling pain-free at the time of the exam.

DOCUMENTING A PAIN ASSESSMENT

Documentation is the final step in a comprehensive pain assessment. It is an important step in communication among the health care team so that the information can be used in planning interventions for pain relief, as well as diagnosing the cause of the pain. Excellent documentation of pain assessment allows the practitioner to evaluate relief measures as well as improvement or decline in the client's condition. An initial pain assessment may be quite lengthy. It can be documented as a narrative note; however, a common framework should be used. It may consist of the assessment framework, such as the head-to-toe method or an independent framework incorporating all aspects of the assessment process. It must include type, severity (or intensity), onset, duration, location, and history of previous pain.

Flow sheets have been developed for pain assessment, incorporating multiple assessments as well as space to document intervention and evaluation. The severity may be documented as a number value if using a standard scale, or a linear or visual analog may be displayed and marked at each pain assessment. Some facilities include an anatomical drawing, front and back, so that the location of the pain can be drawn or indicated (Figure 2-6). Medications used for pain control should be documented, including the dose, route, duration of use, side effects experienced, and the client's view of efficacy. Interventions that are not effective should be discarded.

Pain is not static; it may change often due to multiple factors. For this reason, pain assessments should be done frequently, on a regular basis, and documented clearly and completely. Health care providers should not wait for a client complaint to institute further assessment. It is essential to remember that the client is the very best indicator of pain; pain is what the client describes.

Case Study Resolved

After completing Mr. A.'s assessment, the nurse documents her findings in the chart. The doctor has Mr. A. walk at a moderate pace on a treadmill. Within 6 minutes, Mr. A. complains of bilateral calf pain radiating to the thigh area. He rates it as a "7" on the linear scale. The pain resolves spontaneously after resting for 15 minutes with his legs in a dependent position. Pending further testing, the doctor diagnoses this pain as intermittent claudication, a hallmark symptom of arterial peripheral vascular disease. He will be treated with medication, exercise to promote collateral circulation, and some lifestyle changes. Because this pain is caused by a lack of oxygen to the muscle tissues, the nurse reminds Mr. A. not to use applied heat to the area as a method of pain relief. The heat increases metabolism in the area, increasing the oxygen debt and exacerbating the pain.

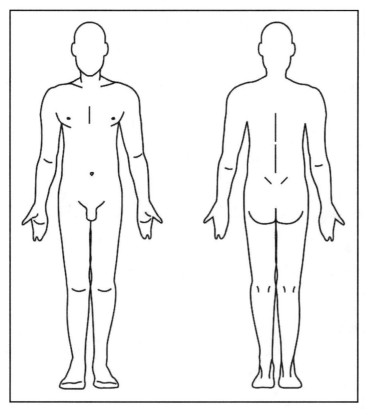

Figure 2-6. Drawings used to determine areas of pain and radiation.

REFERENCE

1. Acute Pain Management Clinical Practice Guideline Panel. *Acute Pain Management: Operative or Medical Procedures and Trauma. AHCPR Pub No. 92-0032.* Rockville, Md: Agency for Health Care Policy and Research, US Department of Health and Human Services, Public Health Service; 1992.

BIBLIOGRAPHY

Ferrell B, Whedon M, Rollins B, et al. Pain and quality assessment/improvement. *J Nurs Care Qual.* 1995;9(3):69-85.

Mayer DD, Torma L, Byock I, Norris K. Speaking the language of pain. *Am J Nurs.* 2001;101(2):44-50.

McCaffery M, Pasero C. *Pain: Clinical Manual.* 2nd ed. St. Louis, Mo: Mosby; 1999.

Torma LA. Pain as the fifth vital sign task force. *Missoula Demonstration Project: The Quality of Life's End.* Available at: http://www.missoulademonstration.org/fifth_vital_sign_tf.shtml. Accessed 2000.

RELATED WEBSITES

The Agency for Healthcare Research and Quality: www.ahrq.gov
The American Academy of Pain Management: www.aapainmanage.org
The American Academy of Pain Medicine: www.painmed.org
The American Chronic Pain Association: www.theacpa.org
The American Pain Foundation: www.painfoundation.org
The American Pain Society: www.ampainsoc.org
The American Society of Pain Management Nurses: www.aspmn.org

MULTIPLE-CHOICE QUESTIONS

1. The most essential step to providing pain management for an individual client is a:
   A. Comprehensive pain assessment
   B. Comprehensive health history
   C. Written plan of care
   D. Familiarity with prescription medications often used for pain control

2. A comprehensive pain assessment includes information concerning:
   A. Type of pain
   B. Duration of pain
   C. Medication history
   D. All of the above

3. Which of the following are potential barriers to pain assessment?
   A. Language and culture
   B. Diet and exercise
   C. Site and duration of pain
   D. Client education

4. The following scale is appropriate to measure pain in the 3-year-old child:
   A. Linear scale marked 1 through 10
   B. A "faces of pain" scale illustrating happy through crying
   C. A linear scale with printed words describing pain
   D. A verbal scale with words describing the pain

5. During a physical assessment for pain, it is important for the nurse to consider that:
   A. Chronic pain and acute pain are frequently expressed in the same manner
   B. Pain is only a subjective phenomenon
   C. There is a characteristic shift in vital signs for all clients in pain
   D. Chronic pain can be expressed very differently from acute pain

6. Functional assessment of the client with pain should include:
   A. The client's ability to complete activities of daily living
   B. The client's willingness to use prescribed remedies
   C. Extended social support for the client
   D. Function of major organ systems

7. Pain assessment should be done:
   A. Only once
   B. Once each shift or visit
   C. By one single caregiver
   D. Repeatedly to assist with managing fluctuations or changes in the client's pain

MULTIPLE-CHOICE ANSWERS

1. A. This assessment includes both subjective and objective data.
2. D. All are important in formulating a plan of care for the client experiencing pain.
3. A. Culture and/or language may affect how pain is expressed.
4. B. is most appropriate, allowing the child to communicate using visual cues. Numbers and words are less appropriate because of developmental level and the potential for developmental regression during pain or illness.
5. D. Individuals with chronic pain may appear very different from those with acute pain.
6. A. Ability to participate in activities of daily living, including self-care and life roles, are part of the functional assessment.
7. D. Continual assessment improves pain management.

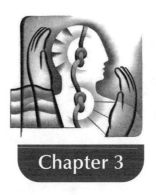

Chapter 3

Interventions for Pain Relief

Case Study

Mrs. P., a 74-year-old woman who is active and in excellent health, states she has pain and swelling in both knees. She describes this as a progressive process, occurring with increasing frequency and severity over the past 6 years. She has used aspirin and sometimes a heating pad as means of pain relief with good success until recently. Over the past 4 months, she states that she has not been able to ride her bike, that kneeling to do her gardening has become impossible, and that even walking has become painful. The aspirin doesn't seem to help anymore.

On physical examination, both knees are swollen, red, and warm to touch. After x-rays and further testing, a diagnosis of severe osteoarthritis is made. Because Mrs. P. is in good health and prefers her previous level of activity, bilateral joint replacement is decided upon. Replacement of the knees will reduce pain and increase Mrs. P.'s ability to return to her previous level of activity.

Once effective assessment of pain is complete, pain management strategies must be identified to promote optimal pain relief. Ways to manage the client's pain may be pharmacological, including analgesics, opioids, and anesthetics. Other options may be physiological, including methods of transcutaneous stimulation, postural changes, or use of acupuncture or acupressure points. Finally, behavioral measures including education, relaxation, guided imagery, or other client choices can be incorporated into the plan. The plan of care may include traditional medical approaches, as well as nontraditional, cultural, or religious variables, which may be identified either by the client or caregiver. It is important in designing the plan of care to include both traditional and nontraditional interventions for optimal relief, rather than take an all-or-none approach. One single intervention rarely provides complete relief for the client. This chapter will provide a review of many of the pain management strategies available, but research continually uncovers new strategies as well as innovative and different ways to utilize old ones.

MEDICATION FOR PAIN RELIEF

Medication is a commonly used and well-respected intervention for pain relief. It is used with or without the participation of a health care provider. The client or client's family may choose an over-the-counter medication perceived as appropriate to the client's symptoms or may choose to use a prescription medication either left over from a previous experience with pain or belonging to someone other than the client. When the client chooses to contact the health care provider for treatment of pain, it is often medication that is expected as an intervention.

Medications to relieve pain include:
- NSAIDs
- COX-2 inhibitors
- Opioids
- Local and regional anesthetics
- Adjuvant medications (eg, antidepressants, anticonvulsants)
- Medications specific to disease or condition

A wide variety of medications are available for pain management. They include commonly used "pain" medications as well as adjuvant medicines, which help to relieve factors that can cause or aggravate pain. Medications that treat the cause of the pain are also instrumental in relieving pain. Medication for specific painful conditions such as angina or neuroleptic pain can be used. Rarely is a single medication successful in alleviating pain unless it is a medicine used to treat pain with a very specific causative factor or the pain is quite mild.

Pain is classified as mild, moderate, or severe.

Pain is usually classified as mild, moderate, or severe. Severity of pain, along with type and location, are parameters used in initially choosing a medication protocol. Common pain medications include nonopioid analgesics and opioids or narcotics. Nonopioids include acetaminophen, salicylates like aspirin, and nonsteroidal anti-inflammatory drugs (NSAIDs) including ibuprofen. These medications, some of which also have antipyretic or anti-inflammatory properties, are chosen to treat mild to moderate pain. With the advent of availability of over-the-counter NSAIDs several years ago (eg, Motrin, Advil), all three of these types of medications are available to clients for self-treatment of mild to moderate pain. One drawback in the use of these medications is dosage scheduling. They may be prescribed by health care professionals or used by clients on a PRN basis, not taken until pain is evident or until discomfort is becoming worse. It becomes more of a challenge to alleviate present pain than to prevent recurrence of pain. For this reason, around-the-clock dosage schedules may be more effective for optimal pain relief.

When possible, an around-the-clock schedule of administration may provide more success with pain relief than administering medication on a PRN basis.

Nonopioids are limited in that they have a ceiling to their doses, beyond which significant toxicity can occur,

Table 3-1

Dosing Data for Oral NSAIDs

Drug	Usual Adult Dose	Usual Pediatric Dose	Comments
Acetaminophen	650–975 mg q 4 hrs	10–15 mg/kg q 4 hrs	Lacks the peripheral anti-inflammatory activity of other NSAIDs
Aspirin	650–975 mg q 4 hrs	10–15 mg/kg q 4 hrs	Standard against which other NSAIDs are compared; inhibits platelet aggregation; may cause postop bleeding
Choline magnesium trisalicylate (Trilisate)	1000–1500 mg BID	25 mg/kg BID	May have minimal antiplatelet activity; also available as oral liquid
Diflunisal (Dolobid)	1000 mg initial dose followed by 500 mg q 12 hrs		
Etodolac (Lodine)	200–400 mg q 6–8 hrs		
Fenoprofen calcium (Nalfon)	200 mg q 4–6 hrs		
Ibuprofen (Motrin, etc)	400 mg q 4–6 hrs	10 mg/kg q 6–8 hrs	Many brand names and generic available; also as oral suspension
Ketoprofen (Orudis)	25–75 mg q 6–8 hrs		
Magnesium salicylate	650 mg q 4 hrs		Many brands and generic forms available

Source: Acute Pain Management Guideline Panel. *Acute Pain Management: Operative or Medical Procedures and Trauma. Clinical Practice Guideline. AHCPR Pub No. 92-0032*. Rockville, Md: Agency for Health Care Policy and Research, Public Health Service, US Department of Health and Human Service; 1992.

presenting danger to the client. Each has its own group of side effects, which should be known and readily recognized by the health care provider who is prescribing their use (Table 3-1). Most medications in these classes are available primarily in oral dose form, however, several are available in suppository form. Several rarely used NSAIDs are available for parenteral administration.

Acetaminophen, aspirin, and NSAIDs are relatively inexpensive, readily available and do not cause central nervous system (CNS)-related side effects such as bowel or bladder problems, sedation, or respiratory depression. NSAIDs, however, can cause gastrointestinal bleeding because they block prostaglandin synthesis and can interfere with the mucosal barrier of the gastrointestinal tract. Because renal function depends on prostaglandins, NSAIDS should also be used cautiously in individuals with impaired renal function. Each year there are approximately 107,000 hospitalizations with more than 16,500 deaths related to side effects of NSAIDs. Individuals at risk for gastrointestinal side effects of NSAIDs may be given COX-2 (cyclo-oxygenase isoenzyme) inhibitors for their analgesic effect. COX-2 inhibitors have a better safety profile than NSAIDs because of their sparing effect on platelet aggregation and on the gastrointestinal tract. As of August 2001, celecoxib (Celebrex, Pharmacia, Peapack, NJ) and rofecoxib (Vioxx, Merck, Whitehouse Station, NJ) are the COX-2 inhibitors prescribed most frequently. Although these COX-2 inhibitors have risk for gastrointestinal bleeding, they too are contraindicated in some client populations. Celecoxib is contraindicated if a client has allergic reactions to sulfonamides. Both celecoxib and rofecoxib are contraindicated in clients who have experienced asthma, urticaria, or allergic reactions after taking aspirin or other NSAIDs.

When pain is moderate to severe or NSAID or COX-2 inhibitor therapy has failed, the addition of an opioid to the treatment plan is indicated. Prior to adding an opioid, review the NSAID's dosage schedule. If PRN dosing was used, it may be possible to have success with NSAIDs administered around the clock. NSAIDs are good potentiators of opioid medication. Opioids work by binding with opioid receptor sites in the central and peripheral nervous systems. Using NSAIDs in combination with opioids usually results in effective pain management with smaller necessary doses of opioids, thereby reducing the CNS side effects associated with opioid use. In addition to CNS side effects, opioids are associated with physical tolerance and psychological dependence. Physical tolerance is unusual in the client with pain using opioids for a short period.

Codeine, oxycodone, morphine, meperidine (Demerol, Sanofi Pharmaceuticals, Paris, France) and hydrocodone are opioids commonly used in pain management. Codeine, oxycodone, and hydrocodone are often used for moderate pain in an oral form in combination with acetaminophen, if tolerated by the client. Oxycodone and hydrocodone are not available in parenteral formulations, so codeine may be chosen for those clients who cannot tolerate oral medication. Clients often report nausea, vomiting, sedation, and feelings of "disconnectedness" with these medications. If one of these medications causes unpleasant side effects such as nausea, the client may be able to tolerate one of the others. Codeine and the codeine derivatives are frequently prescribed as pain therapy following outpatient invasive procedures, including diagnostics and dental surgery. They are inexpensive and come in combination tablet form with NSAIDs. It is important to be aware of the ceiling dose of the combined NSAID when titrating medication dosages upward for pain relief.

Morphine sulfate and hydromorphone (Dilaudid) are more commonly used for severe pain or after procedures when it is expected that severe pain will occur. These medications are often administered parenterally, but addition of an NSAID when the client can tolerate oral medication may increase comfort and decrease the need for opioids. Meperidine is another medication used after procedures, but it is not recommended in elders or in clients with renal dysfunction. If meperidine is given parenterally, it should only be used for 48 hours because of the risk of normeperidine toxicity.

When meperidine is prescribed, doses should be adequate to provide good pain relief. It is often prescribed in inadequate doses. Intravenous meperidine has a short serum half-life.

Morphine sulfate is the "gold standard" for opioid pain relief. It is against this standard that dosing and efficacy are measured and equianalgesic tables are constructed. It is available in oral, parenteral, and rectal preparations, as well as in immediate-release and extended-release oral forms. Clients using morphine may experience nausea and vomiting, which usually resolves within 24 hours of the first dose and is responsive to conventional antiemetic therapy. Itching is another unpleasant side effect described by a small percentage of clients who use morphine. Inability to provide comfort from these side effects requires consideration of a different opioid for pain relief.

In addition to sedation and respiratory depression, opioids can cause constipation, which can have a significantly negative impact on quality of life. Baseline bowel assessment should be done, with continued assessment for regular bowel activity during opioid use. Addition of extra fluids and extra fiber to the diet or a bulk laxative with adequate fluid intake should be instituted when the client can tolerate it. Untreated constipation related to opioid use will increase a client's level of discomfort.

Efficacy of opioid use depends on assessment for pain relief, as well as the presence of medication side effects. Poor relief in the absence of side effects allows for increased doses of the opioid. Other medications that enhance the activity of the opioid or reduce factors that cause or exacerbate pain should also be considered for use. These are called adjuvant medications—drugs used in addition to the already prescribed therapy. Use of adjuvant medications does not preclude the NSAIDs previously incorporated into the opioid regimen. Potentiators of opioids include benzodiazapines and phenothiazines. Anti-anxiety medications such as diazepam (Valium) or lorazepam (Ativan, Wyeth, Philadelphia, Pa) promote relaxation, may reduce muscular tension, and reduce anxiety. Lorazepam and antihistamines also act as antiemetics, reducing nausea and vomiting. Diphenhydramine (Benadryl, Pfizer, New York, NY), a common antihistamine, when used with morphine can help to relieve nausea and itching. Steroids reduce inflammation. It is important to consider undesirable side effects like increased sedation, which may also be enhanced by the adjuvant medications.

Finally, certain medications are specific to certain pain syndromes. Neuroleptic or nerve pain is not well-relieved with the use of opioids, and the pain is often too severe to respond solely to anti-inflammatory therapy. Phantom pain following amputation or pain from nerve compression by tumor or fracture are two good examples of this type of pain. Tricyclic antidepressants and anticonvulsant medications are much more useful in relieving this type of pain. Cardiac anginal pain, which occurs as the result of inadequate oxygen to the myocardium, responds to morphine partly because the sedating effect reduces cardiac metabolism, also reducing the oxygen deficit. Vasodilators are successfully used to relieve anginal pain, both cardiac and elsewhere in the body, by increasing circulation and oxygen delivery to the affected area. Local anesthetic agents are used topically or subcutaneously for local pain control.

Choice and administration of medications include considering the "five rights" in client-focused safety: the right drug, the right dose, the right time, the right route, and the right

> The "five rights" for safety are:
> 1. The right drug
> 2. The right dose
> 3. The right time
> 4. The right route
> 5. The right client

client. Choosing an appropriate route for medication administration takes into consideration many factors. Oral medication is commonly the easiest and most cost-effective route of choice. It is appropriate when the client can safely swallow and tolerate oral intake. When oral administration is not an option, less invasive routes include sublingual, rectal, and transcutaneous, as dictated by the availability of medication for that particular route. Subcutaneous injection allows for deposit and absorption of small volumes of fluid; intramuscular injection will accommodate larger volumes, but still no more than 2.5 cc. Intravenous injection of medication allows for larger volumes of fluid as well as extremely rapid delivery. Medication administered intravenously has a shorter half-life within the body, because it is more rapidly delivered to the liver and kidneys for clearance from the body. Intravenous delivery of opioids is potentially more dangerous because of the risk of overdose. The antidote naloxone (Narcan, DuPont Pharma, Madrid, Spain) should be readily available to completely block opioid action in case of accidental overdose when the intravenous route is used.

Intravenous administration of opioids is the route of choice when a PCA (patient-controlled analgesia) pump is used in the plan of care. The PCA pump allows the client to use a button to make the pump inject a predetermined dose of medication into an IV. Maximum dose over a determined time frame is programmed into the pump computer, preventing the client from receiving any more medication than has been ordered. It is a safe and effective way of promoting client involvement in pain management, allowing client control over the medication. This alternative is more comfortable for clients than repeated intermittent injections and is cost-effective, reducing nursing time spent with multiple intermittent administrations. Sophisticated pump computers allow the health care provider to track how frequently medication is requested by the client and whether a dose was delivered or not. The client who can use a PCA pump must be motivated to use the equipment, be able to learn how to use it, be available for client education, and be a candidate for IV administration of an opioid. Side effects of the opioid can certainly occur with use of a PCA pump. Oversedation is rare, because as the client becomes more sedated, requests for medication become less frequent. Other side effects such as nausea, itching, and confusion should be addressed right away using conventional interventions or a change in medication. PCA pumps can be programmed to deliver a bolus of medication as requested, simulating a PRN dose schedule; or a basal rate of medication can be programmed for continuous infusion, with smaller boluses available for breakthrough pain or to increase activity tolerance, as requested by the client. To promote optimal relief of pain, NSAIDs or COX-2 inhibitors are often used in conjunction with opioid therapy NSAIDs.

EQUIANALGESIC PAIN MANAGEMENT

When pain management is effective but it is necessary to change medication or route, an equianalgesic chart should be consulted so that the client will not be over- or under-medicated using the new route or medication. An excellent example of the need for a change, despite successful pain relief, is when a surgical client who is maintained comfortably on the PCA pump is changed to oral (PO) medication in preparation for discharge home. It is vital to keep this client comfortable, to enable increased mobility, and to return to baseline activities of daily living. By identifying the amount of medication the client is currently receiving, a comparable amount of the new medication can be ordered. Even a change in route only requires reference to the equianalgesic table. The table uses morphine as the standard, and comparable amounts of other medications and their routes are listed. The chart provides a guideline for initial dosing when making a change in drug and/or route (Table 3-2). For example, a client receiving morphine sulfate 3 mg IV every 3 hours for adequate pain control will be changed to Percocet (oxycodone 5 mg and acetaminophen 325 mg) in preparation for discharge home. He has used Percocet with good effect in the past. Referring to the equianalgesic chart, the health care provider will order two Percocet tablets (oxycodone 10 mg and acetaminophen 650 mg) to be taken every 4 hours. The client's pain relief will then be evaluated on this new medication, with revisions made to the plan before discharge home.

Case Study Revisited

Upon return at 1:00 pm to the postoperative floor after uncomplicated replacement of her right knee, Mrs. P. has morphine sulfate 2 to 3 mg SC q 2-3 hours PRN ordered for pain. She complains of moderate to severe pain throughout the afternoon, describing it as 7 on a scale of 1 to 10. She requests medication every 2 hours. By 6:00 pm she is unable to tolerate her evening meal because of intense feelings of nausea. Her primary nurse realizes that it will be a long, uncomfortable night unless some changes are made in the plan of care.

A conversation with the surgeon results in new medication orders: meperidine (Demerol) 50 mg with hydroxyzine hydrochloride (Vistaril) 50 mg IM q 4 hours around the clock for pain. The nurse believes that this client would have been a good candidate for a PCA pump but has had no training to use one and is now too uncomfortable. She gives Mrs. P. her first shot of Demerol and Vistaril, explaining that the Vistaril not only makes the Demerol more effective but will help decrease the nausea. Mrs. P. reports feeling much more comfortable within the space of 1 hour.

The nurse also does some simple relaxation exercises with her, primarily controlled breathing and progressive muscle relaxation, and helps her to change her position in bed. By 10:30 pm, Mrs. P. is sleeping, but the night nurse will be careful to continue to administer the IM pain medication even if the client is asleep to prevent the recurrence of severe pain.

PHYSICAL STRATEGIES TO MANAGE PAIN

Manipulation and change in the client's physical status present another variety of pain control techniques. These are useful as adjuvant therapies in moderate to severe pain or may sometimes be used alone when pain is mild or medication is poorly tolerated. Some of these strategies may be performed independently, while others may require the assistance of another.

> It is important when presenting physical and behavioral alternatives to clients to discuss them as complementary therapies. If the client perceives the strategies as an absolute replacement for medication, then pain management may fail.

Touch is a simple strategy used in caring for the client in pain. Touch can provide reassurance, a sense of contact and involvement, and may facilitate relaxation. Muscular tension can be a causative factor for some types of pain or may be a contributing factor in others. Promoting reduced tension can assist with pain relief. Other types of cutaneous or

Table 3-2

Dose Equivalents for Opioid Analgesics in Opioid-Naive Clients ≥ 50 kg Body Weight*

Drug	Approximate Equianalgesic Dose		Usual Starting Dose for Moderate to Severe Pain	
	Oral	Parenteral	Oral	Parenteral
Opioid Agonist**				
Morphine	30 mg q 3–4 hrs (repeat around-the-clock dosing) 60 mg q 3–4 hrs (single or intermittent dosing)	10 mg q 3–4 hrs	30 mg q 3–4 hrs	10 mg q 3–4 hrs
Morphine, controlled release (MS Contin, Ora-Morph)	90–120 mg q 12 hrs	N/A	90–120 mg q 12 hrs	N/A
Hydromorphone (Dilaudid)	7.5 mg q 3–4 hrs	1.5 mg q 3–4 hrs	6 mg q 3–4 hrs	1.5 mg q 3–4 hrs
Levorphanol (Levo-Dromoran)	4 mg q 6–8 hrs	2 mg q 6–8 hrs	4 mg q 6–8 hrs	2 mg q 6–8 hrs
Meperidine (Demerol)	300 mg q 2–3 hrs	100 mg q 3 hrs	N/R	100 mg q 3 hrs
Methadone (Dolophine, etc)	20 mg q 6–8 hrs	10 mg q 6–8 hrs	20 mg q 6–8 hrs	10 mg q 6–8 hrs
Oxymorphone (Numorphan)	N/A	1 mg q 3–4 hrs	N/A	1 mg q 3–4 hrs
Combination Opioid/NSAID Preparations+				
Codeine (with aspirin or acetaminophen)	180–200 mg q 3–4 hrs	130 mg q 3–4 hrs	60 mg q 3–4 hrs	60 mg q 2 hrs (IM/SC)
Hydrocodone (in Lorcet, Lortab, Vicodin, etc)	30 mg q 3–4 hrs	N/A	10 mg q 3–4 hrs	N/A
Oxycodone (Roxicodone, also in Percocet, Percodan, Tylox, etc)	30 mg q 3–4 hrs	N/A	10 mg q 3–4 hrs	N/A

*Caution: Recommended doses do not apply for adults with body weight < 50 kg.
**Caution: Recommended doses do not apply to clients with renal or hepatic insufficiency or other conditions affecting drug metabolism and kinetics.
+Caution: For these drugs, rectal administration is an alternate route for patients unable to take oral medications.

Source: Acute Pain Management Guideline Panel. *Acute Pain Management: Operative or Medical Procedures and Trauma. Clinical Practice Guideline.* AHCPR Pub No. 92-0032. Rockville, Md: Agency for Health Care Policy and Research, Public Health Service, US Department of Health and Human Service; 1992.

transcutaneous stimulation can also be used in pain relief. *Gentle cutaneous stimulation,* either at the site of pain or at another site on the body, can have the effect of confounding the gate control for pain stimulus, short circuiting the system and reducing the perceived painful sensations. This light, rhythmic stroking with only a feather-light touch is called *effleurage.* It is often taught to pregnant women for use in labor pain management. It can be performed by a caregiver or by the client himself.

Massage is another form of touch that can be gentle or more vigorous. Gentle massage, in which stroking is rhythmic but not as light as effleurage, can reduce pain gate sensations or help to promote muscle relaxation. Deep massage, usually done by a health care provider or massage therapist, promotes relaxation and a sense of well-being but should be used only in specific situations. Clients with bleeding dyscrasias or who are at risk for clot or thrombus formation are not candidates for massage. These clients are at risk for bleeding, bruising, or embolization with massage. One good example is a client with leg pain as the result of a deep vein thrombosis. Massage is especially beneficial for the client with chronic pain. *Reflexology* is an ancient form of natural healing that uses massage at reflex points on the feet. Specific points refer to specific body areas and will promote relief from pain and healing in that area.

> In order to avoid unnecessary risk of injury, massage for a client with health problems should only be done by a trained professional who is familiar with the client's specific condition.

Application of *heat or cold therapy* is another form of cutaneous or transcutaneous stimulation that may add to pain relief. Application of cold to the painful area results in slight numbing. The sensation of cold is sent as a message to the central nervous system, short-circuiting the gate control mechanism for pain. Decrease in local body temperature results in slight vasoconstriction of the area, reducing local circulation as well as limiting the amount of extracellular fluid leaking into the area. Limiting extracellular fluid reduces or prevents swelling. Swelling, through increased local pressure, may increase or even be a cause of pain. It is important when using application of cold to relieve pain to protect the skin. Ice should not be applied directly, rather it should be wrapped in a towel or cloth. Cold should be applied intermittently. A good rule is 20 minutes on—20 minutes off. Continuous application of cold could result in tissue damage as the result of continued vasoconstriction.

Use of heat in pain relief is another common choice. Warmth promotes muscular relaxation and a sense of comfort. As previously noted, decreasing muscular tension may reduce pain sensations. Vasodilatation occurs locally in the area where heat is applied. This increases circulation, enhancing the removal of cellular debris, toxins, and extracellular fluid from the area of tissue injury. Although heat is not useful in preventing swelling, it is a great aid in reducing swelling that has already occurred. Reduction in swelling may enhance comfort. As with the application of cold, care should be taken to protect the skin where heat is applied. The older client, or one with neuropathy, is at risk for burns when heat injury is not noticed. Clients with mental status changes or who are sedated should not use heat for pain relief without supervision, as injury may result. Continuous application of heat is contraindicated for a variety of reasons. The same 20 on—20 off rule, as used when applying cold, is a good idea. Temperature of any heating device should be frequently checked to prevent burns. Finally, heat should never be applied to an area where arterial vascular insufficiency is suspected. In this instance, metabolism and oxygen need are increased, putting the client in danger of injury from oxygen deficit.

Change in position may also facilitate pain reduction. A new position can relieve pressure over bony prominences or areas of swelling. It can promote increased circulation, muscle relaxation, and general comfort. The client in pain may be reluctant to change position, fearing that pain will increase or damage will be done. Immobility as the result of pain can cause multiple complications. It is important to teach the client how to change position safely and comfortably. Aids in changing position such as an overhead trapeze, bed rails, or arms on a chair are helpful. Use of pain medication or other adjuvant therapies prior to position change can further reduce discomfort.

Exercise as a method of pain control is being investigated. Exercise, even gentle exercise, results in the release of endorphins, the body's own opioids. Endorphin release promotes natural pain reduction, as well as feelings of well-being. Exercise is also helpful in changing muscle tension, encouraging repositioning, and promoting increased function, such as when the client ambulates after abdominal surgery, resulting in an increase in intestinal peristalsis.

Therapeutic touch and *reiki* are energy-based approaches to pain relief. Therapeutic touch uses the body's energy to promote relaxation and pain relief. Reiki promotes bodily, emotional, and spiritual harmony through precise hand placement on the client's body, resulting in increased pain relief. Both of these therapies promote a sense of warmth and well-being.

Acupuncture and *acupressure* are ancient Eastern techniques that involve changing energy flow through meridian or energy lines mapped throughout the body. Acupuncture involves the insertion of fine needles into identified acupuncture points, promoting balance and relief from pain. It requires the participation of a trained acupuncture practitioner. Insertion of the needles causes little or no discomfort. Acupressure involves exerting gentle continuous or intermittent pressure over identified pressure points, altering energy flow and promoting pain relief. It can be done by a health care professional or by the client after specific points have been identified and pressure techniques taught. Acupressure is also used in managing concurrent symptoms, such as when nausea is a problematic side effect of pain medication.

Aromatherapy utilizes scents from essential oils to promote relaxation and relieve symptoms. Specific essential oils have specific uses, such as lavender for relaxation and tension reduction or ginger for nausea relief. The oil is placed in very small amounts on cotton or at strategic places in the environment. It can be used in health care facilities and taught to the client for independent use at home. This treatment modality is presently receiving much study.

Cultural alternatives including the use of herbal remedies, cultural healers or practitioners, religious rituals such as prayer, and specific alternatives that have worked very successfully in the past should be incorporated into the plan of care. The health care provider can gain awareness of these methods through learning about the cultures or religions of clients served in a specific geographical area and through careful history-taking and assessment of the client and family. It is very important to be aware of the type of herbal remedies a client is using, as certain substances may enhance or inhibit medications being used, resulting in a change in the efficacy of these medications or presenting risks to the client.

Transcutaneous electric nerve stimulation (TENS) involves passing a mild electric current across the skin to superficial nerves near the location of the pain. Electrodes with positive and negative poles are placed on the skin and a current flows intermittently across them, providing pain relief. Relief is temporary but recurs with repeated current stimulation. A small battery-powered generator is used to provide electric current. This strategy for pain relief is initially set up by a health care provider but is usually controlled by the client and can be used in almost any setting. Despite the cost of equipment, it is cost-efficient and safe, although some clients are reluctant to use electric current for therapy. It is especially useful in treating chronic pain conditions.

BEHAVIORAL STRATEGIES FOR PAIN RELIEF

Behavioral strategies include intellectual, emotional, and psychosocial approaches to pain management. Their use can be extremely effective with a motivated client (and health caregiver) who is open to trying these somewhat unconventional methods.

Relaxation is a combination of physical and behavior methods. It can be achieved through controlled breathing exercises, *visual or guided imagery*, or progressive muscle relaxation. Relaxation reduces physical and emotional tension and promotes the release of endorphins. It also helps the client to feel more in control of the situation. Meditation is a controlled, focused flow of thought that may also have a relaxing effect on the client and, through focus, help him or her to be more in control. *Meditation* is a learned skill; considerable client education and practice is necessary for success. Biofeedback is a means of measuring muscular tension, electrical stimulation across the skin, and/or respiratory rate. *Biofeedback* provides concrete information to the client about his or her state of relaxation or arousal. Through successful use of biofeedback, the client can be more successful in reducing tension and anxiety.

Guided imagery can be useful not only in promoting relaxation, but in actual pain relief as well. Visualization of a special place such as the beach or mountainside is used in relaxation and as distraction from discomfort. Proactive pain relief with guided imagery uses the imagination or an imaginary device to reduce pain. One strategy is to have the client visualize a meter and allow the meter to indicate present level of pain. It is a good idea not to become too elaborate in requesting the client to visualize this meter. Rather, allow the client to elaborate on what type of meter it is, having him or her describe it at length.

Then, through imagery, the client turns down the level of pain on the meter, translating to less actual pain. Clients who practice this technique repeatedly can become quite successful. It is very useful for the client who must undergo repeated painful procedures.

Hypnosis and *self-hypnosis* have been used successfully in pain management. A trained hypnotherapist can place the client in a suggestible state and in this state help the client to manage pain or other adverse symptoms. It is very important for the client to understand that during hypnosis an individual cannot be forced to do something or divulge information. Not all clients are candidates for hypnosis. Those who resist it or are fearful of it and its consequences, even after receiving detailed information, should not be considered for this intervention. Clients can be trained to induce their own hypnotic state through self-hypnosis and to use this state of relaxation and focus to help reduce unpleasant symptoms.

Distraction from painful stimuli can be very successful in many client populations. Distraction can include simple interventions such as company, conversation, reading or television, or uncomplicated tasks. Distraction may also include participation in some ADLs. For example, many clients who are employed may bring work with them to treatment facilities. It is not unusual to see a client working on a laptop computer at the bedside. Engagement in activity provides distraction from pain.

Music therapy is a method consisting of active or passive use of music. There is evidence that music therapy can induce relaxation, moderate mood, and result in reduction of pain. Allowing the client to choose the type of music may increase success.

> An elderly man in an oncology clinic chose to bring a recording of hula music on all of his visits. During uncomfortable procedures he would "go to Hawaii." By using his own combination of music therapy and guided imagery, he was successful in managing pain.

Music can be played in the environment or through earphones for only the client to hear. This has become a common practice during dental procedures. Some clients dislike the sense of isolation they get from wearing headphones, because they are then unable to hear what is going on around them.

Humor is an excellent alternative in managing pain. The act of laughing helps to generate endorphins and promote muscular relaxation. It can help reduce anxiety as well. Humor must be appropriate and not offensive. The client must be open and receptive to attempts at humor. Many facilities have instituted the use of *humor carts*, which contain humorous books, videos, collections of cartoons, and sometimes even samples of clients' own writings. Humor carts enable the clients to use this intervention on their own. When clients are part of a group, such as in an ambulatory treatment center or a long-term treatment facility, humor can become part of the group dynamic, used as a way to facilitate coping.

None of the behavioral therapies can be used successfully without *client education*. For this reason, adjuvant therapies have become the domain of the nurse as client educator. A plan for education, as well as assessment of learning styles and skills, for each individual client is necessary. Information in a variety of formats will enhance learning, as will multiple education sessions. Evaluation of material learned and reinforcement sessions will also enhance success.

> When providing client education, it is important to remember that pain is definitely a barrier to learning!

Through creative combinations specifically designed for each individual client, pharmacological, physical, and behavioral strategies can be effectively used for optimal pain relief. Client satisfaction with treatment and its effect on pain should always be the goal, and factors such as cost or health provider attitudes should never be barriers to care. Unfortunately, barriers such as cost and attitudes of health care providers can interfere with treatment of pain. Reimbursement for analgesics in health maintenance organizations (HMOs) is often limited to a few analgesics or NSAIDs. If these medications are effective and do not present a significant risk to a client, they may be appropriate. But medications on third-party formularies should not put a client at risk for a significant side effect or limit the potential effect the client could achieve with a drug that is not on the formulary because of cost. In short, cost should never be the determining factor for choice of treatment for pain. Health care providers also need to consider optimal treatment plans without adding additional burdens. For example, analgesics such as acetaminophen and some NSAIDs are not available by prescription; therefore, they are not covered by most insurance plans. Despite the fact that they are not particularly expensive, lack of insurance coverage may make them an extravagance to some clients. It is vitally important to assess resource availability when suggesting use of an over-the-counter medication or any drug that is not covered by a client's insurance policy.

Case Study Resolved

By the third postoperative day, Mrs. P. is ambulating with the assistance of a walker. Her pain is well controlled with two Percocet (oxycodone 5 mg and acetaminophen 325 mg) tablets taken PRN every 6 hours. She is careful to request them at least 20 minutes before she expects the physical therapist to come. She mentions to the nurse that she has not had a bowel movement since before surgery. A bulk fiber laxative is administered, and the nurse instructs her to drink at least eight glasses of fluid each day. Her constipation resolves.

Mrs. P. is discharged to home on postoperative day 6. On a follow-up visit with her surgeon, she reports that her pain improved dramatically right after she returned home. "I think it was because I was so busy," she says. Three months after her surgery, she is completely pain-free in her right knee and has achieved full range of motion. She is anticipating replacement surgery for the left knee in several months time. Her surgeon plans to have her use a PCA pump for pain management directly after surgery.

BIBLIOGRAPHY

Acute Pain Management Guideline Panel. *Acute Pain Management: Operative or Medical Procedures and Trauma. AHCPR Pub No. 92-0032.* Rockville, Md: Agency for Health Care Policy and Research, Public Health Service, US Department of Health and Human Services; 1992.

American Cancer Society. *Complementary and Alternative Cancer Methods.* Atlanta, Ga: Author; 2000.

American College of Rheumatology Committee on Clinical Guidelines. ACR *Guidelines for Osteoarthritis.* Atlanta, Ga: Author; 2000.

Brant JM. Opioid equianalgesic conversion: the right dose. *Clinical Journal of Oncology Nursing.* 2001;5(4):163-165.

Karch AM. *2002 Lippincott's Nursing Drug Guide.* Philadelphia, Pa: Lippincott; 2001.

Kuhn MA. *Complementary Therapies for Health Care Providers.* Philadelphia, Pa: Lippincott; 1999.

Management of Cancer Pain Guideline Panel. *Management of Cancer Pain Clinical Practice Guideline. AHCPR Pub No. 94-0592.* Rockville, Md: Agency for Health Care Policy and Research, Public Health Service, US Department of Health and Human Services; 1994.

McCaffery M, Pasero C. *Pain: Clinical Manual.* 2nd ed. St. Louis, Mo: Mosby; 1999.

National Center for Complementary and Alternative Medicine. *NCCAM Clearinghouse Publication X-42.* Silver Springs, Md: National Institutes of Health; 2000.

Singh G. *Am J Med.* 1998;105(suppl1B):31S-38S.

LEARNING RESOURCE

Sierzant TL, Portu JB, Belgrade MJ, et al. *Pain Management: An Interactive CD-ROM for Clinical Staff Development.* Frederick, Md: Aspen; 2001.

MULTIPLE-CHOICE QUESTIONS

1. The most essential step in providing interventions for pain is:
   A. Medication administration
   B. Comprehensive assessment
   C. Client teaching
   D. Insurance coverage for palliative care

2. When selecting a medication for pain intervention, it is important to consider:
   A. That all medications work for all types of pain
   B. That narcotics or opioids are a better choice to relieve severe pain
   C. That choice of medication includes type, severity, and location of pain, as well as client-specific issues
   D. That medication is always the best choice to ensure relief

3. When utilizing opioids for pain management, it is important to also assess the client's:
   A. Heart rate
   B. Orthostatic blood pressure
   C. Bowel status
   D. Appetite

4. Use of multiple medications together in an attempt to provide pain relief is:
   A. Contraindicated because of multiple side effects
   B. Currently in experimental trials
   C. Useful only for severe acute pain
   D. Used when medications act in a synergistic fashion

5. The primary mechanism of opioids is:
   A. To promote sleep throughout the painful episode
   B. To bind with opioid receptors in the nervous system, blocking pain messages
   C. To promote muscular relaxation, reducing painful stimuli
   D. To induce amnesia, so the client will forget the painful episode

6. The most significant toxicity or side effect for which it is necessary to assess while managing pain with opioids is:
   A. Restlessness
   B. Respiratory depression
   C. Confusion
   D. Tachycardia

7. Neuropathic pain such as phantom pain after amputation is frequently responsive to which type of medication for relief?
   A. NSAIDs
   B. Opioids
   C. Nitrates
   D. Anticonvulsants

8. When considering a change from one type of narcotic medication to another for pain management, the nurse should consider:
   A. Equianalgesia
   B. Bioavailability
   C. Preferred route
   D. Equal dosing

9. The "gold standard" medication on equianalgesic charts to provide comparison is:
   A. Acetaminophen
   B. Morphine
   C. Codeine
   D. Meperidine

10. When planning for equianalgesia, which of the following must be considered:
    A. Medication to be administered
    B. Medication and route of administration
    C. Medication, route of administration, and times of administration
    D. Medication, route of administration, times of administration, and cost to the facility

11. A PCA pump would be an appropriate choice for which client:
    A. A 62-year-old woman with an elective joint replacement
    B. A 5-year-old having a tonsillectomy
    C. A 35-year-old having emergency vascular surgery
    D. A 62-year-old client with Alzheimer's disease

12. The client complaining of abdominal pain related to constipation would most benefit from:
    A. Opioid therapy
    B. Transcutaneous stimulation
    C. Dietary manipulation
    D. Ambulation

MULTIPLE-CHOICE ANSWERS

1. B. Intervention for pain relief cannot begin until a comprehensive assessment is completed.
2. C. Choice of medication for pain relief is dependent on multiple factors.
3. C. Opioids commonly slow intestinal peristalsis, contributing to constipation.
4. D. Multiple medications are used for both acute and chronic pain in an attempt to address multiple causes of the pain as well as providing enhanced effects through synergy.
5. C. Opioids bind with opioid receptor sites, blocking transmission of pain messages to the central nervous system.
6. B. Respiratory depression may occur with opioid use, resulting in a life-threatening oxygen deficit.
7. D. Anticonvulsants disrupt the afferent messages of pain.
8. A. Equianalgesia to prevent under- or overmedication.
9. B. Morphine is the "gold standard" for comparison.
10. C. Medication, route, and half-life of the drug all affect the choice when a different medication is chosen for pain relief.
11. A. This client would most benefit from PCA pain relief because of the opportunity for preoperative instruction on appropriate use.
12. D. Ambulation promotes the increase of peristalsis and the release of flatus, reducing discomfort.

Chapter 4

Acute Pain in the Adult Client

Case Study

Mr. B., a 52-year-old electrical engineer, is admitted at 8:00 pm to the orthopedic unit of a major teaching facility with a closed fracture of the right femur as the result of a bicycle accident. He is awake and alert, and complaining of severe pain in his right leg. He is placed in Buck's traction to temporarily immobilize the area and attempt to reduce muscle spasms. Surgery for open reduction and internal fixation is scheduled for the next morning, so the client is maintained NPO throughout the night. His pain is initially treated with intramuscular meperidine (Demerol), with fair relief.

Acute pain is a frequent problem in the adult population. Acuity, in this case, refers to duration of the pain, not the severity. This is an important factor to share with the adult client, as the word *acute* is synonymous with threatening or severe for many people.

Acute pain in the adult is commonly pain that is problematic for no more than 6 months.[1] Pain continuing past this point is considered chronic, necessitating other treatment alternatives than those used to manage acute pain. In some cases, when the source of pain is identified, the pain may be diagnosed as chronic from the outset because it is the result of a chronic condition, such as rheumatoid arthritis. In other cases, the duration of the pain determines acuity.

> **Acute pain:** pain that occurs as the result of trauma, tissue injury, or illness. This pain lasts or is expected to last for no more than 6 months.
> **Chronic pain:** pain that lasts for longer than 6 months or is expected to last longer than 6 months because it is related to a chronic illness or condition.

Acute pain in the adult has multiple causes, manifestations, and is managed in many different settings. Self-management is common for the adult client with minor to moderate acute pain. Access to professional treatment usually occurs with increased severity of pain, accompanying issues such as open trauma, or when the pain interferes with everyday life.

One frequent causative factor in acute pain is *trauma*. A traumatic event can be work- or leisure-related. It can be as minor as an abrasion as the result of a fall or affect multiple systems such as trauma from a major auto accident. Severity of pain is not necessarily correlated to the type or severity of the traumatic event. Superficial injuries that occur as the result of trauma are frequently associated with severe pain because of the large number of nociceptors present in superficial tissues. First- and second-degree burns are by far more painful for the client than a more severe and destructive third-degree burn, because the third-degree burn or full-thickness injury destroys many of the nociceptors that would send pain messages to the central nervous system. Visceral pain can also result from trauma, including trauma as the result of violence. *Somatic pain* is frequently reported, such as in a fracture or a sprain. Somatic pain is often associated with sports and physical activity.

Multiple examples of acute pain exist in the adult population. Headaches are common in this client population. Headaches may be related to tension, hormonal shifts, and migraines. Sinus inflammation or seasonal allergies are implicated in episodes of acute headaches. Headache pain is also described in certain individuals with a history of multiple or cluster headaches as acute episodes of a chronic condition. Dental pain is another acute complaint in this group. It may precede or be the result of dental surgery.

Medical reasons for acute pain in adults include cardiac and gastric disorders as the most common. In these instances, pain acts as a signal that there is impending or actual damage to the system. Pain related to a medical condition ranges from minor to severe, with no correlation to severity of disease or damage. It is very important for the health care provider to remember that pain is a subjective entity. One client may be incapacitated by pain related to gastrointestinal flu because the pain is perceived as severe, while a different client may continue to function in normal everyday activities through an acute inflammation of the appendix resulting in rupture. Although people often relate cancer to pain, pain is not commonly an early warning sign of cancer; rather, it is more commonly a later symptom of advanced disease.

Pregnancy and childbirth are responsible for acute pain but will not be addressed further in this chapter. Hormonal changes in females can be correlated with acute episodes of pain, including menstrual pain as well as midcycle pain associated with ovulation.

The health care provider has the opportunity to care for the adult client with acute pain in a wide variety of settings. Clients experiencing surgical pain are seen in inpatient and outpatient facilities, including ambulatory surgical clinics, private offices, and at dental offices. Those with medical conditions are seen over the same wide variety of care settings. Long-term care facilities provide services for these clients as well. Most commonly, the adult client with acute pain is ambulatory and at least partly involved in self-care, taking active efforts toward pain relief. Health care access is sought when pain becomes a barrier to activities of daily living (ADLs). It is important to plan care and institute management with the input of each individual client, including him or her in providing for pain relief.

Interventions for Acute Pain

Managing acute pain in the adult client can include pharmacological, physiological, and behavioral interventions. Except for mild pain, strategies for pain relief should include more than one treatment modality for optimal relief.

Types of intervention for acute pain:
- Pharmacological
- Physiological
- Behavioral

Pharmacological choices may be over-the-counter, self-prescribed or self-administered medications, or narcotics with or without the addition of adjunct medications. Careful assessment of the pain for location, type, and severity is necessary prior to instituting relief measures. The clinical guidelines published by the US Department of Health and Human Services offer a step-wise guide to the use of medication for acute pain. Mild to moderate pain may be relieved with the use of nonsteroidal anti-inflammatory drugs (NSAIDs) or other anti-inflammatory agents such as salicylates. These medications in common dosages can be administered on an as-needed (PRN) or around-the-clock basis. Using medication on an as-needed protocol sometimes results in increased severity of pain and reduction in relief, because the medication is not used frequently enough or not used until the pain becomes quite severe. Complications or factors that may make pain worse, such as anxiety or muscular tension, may increase when there are long intervals between doses of medication used on a PRN basis, reducing the effectiveness of simple relief measures. Acute pain of more than a transitory nature may be relieved more effectively by using an NSAID on a regular dosage schedule, rather than waiting to re-experience pain before taking more medication.

Administration schedules for pain medication and adjuvant medications:
- **PRN:** medication is given at minimum hourly parameters upon the assessment by the caregiver that the client has pain or at the client's request (eg, oxycodone and acetaminophen [Percocet], two tablets every 4 to 6 hours, PRN).
- **Around-the-clock:** medication given at determined or ordered hourly intervals throughout the day (eg, oxycodone and acetaminophen [Percocet], two tablets every 6 hours).

Acute pain that is not adequately relieved by these medications on a scheduled dosage protocol, or acute pain that is expected to be more severe such as postsurgical pain, can be treated with the addition of a narcotic. Choice of narcotic will include information about severity of pain, as well as client history of medication use and allergies. Codeine or oxycodone are common choices for less severe pain; morphine or meperidine (Demerol) may be used for pain that is more severe or not well-relieved by codeine or a codeine derivative. Routes of administration for narcotics are also considered. Oral medication is appropriate for the client who is able to tolerate food or fluids. Intravenous medication is useful when the client must be maintained NPO (nothing by mouth), cannot tolerate oral food or fluids, or if extremely rapid relief is vital. Intravenous medications are cleared from the body much more rapidly than other routes, so administration must be more frequent to maintain adequate pain relief. Intramuscular, subcutaneous, or rectal routes are other alternatives. Transcutaneous administration is less commonly used for clients with acute pain. In clients who can tolerate oral medication, the addition of an NSAID to the narcotic regimen will increase efficacy. Oral preparations of codeine and oxycodone are manufactured in a form already in combination with acetaminophen (eg, Tylenol #2, Tylenol #3, or Tylenol #4, and Percocet). One drawback of these combination tablets is that doses can only be titrated as high as the ceiling dose for acetaminophen. If further amounts of narcotic are necessary, plain codeine or oxycodone should be used. Overdoses of acetaminophen can result in liver damage.

Routes of administration may directly affect self-administration in the adult client. Ease of administration, as well as the client's acceptability of the route, are important to consider when planning care. Self-injection or relying on a family member to administer injections may be unacceptable. Many clients object to rectal administration as well, and family members often consider it undignified to administer rectal medications (eg, suppositories). Timed release oral medications, which restrict doses to two or three times per day, decrease client burden and increase client adherence with multiple dose schedules. Ascertaining that the client is comfortable with, understands, and is able to accomplish administration via a prescribed route is essential to client acceptance with a pain management plan.

In addition to narcotics and NSAIDs, other adjuvant medications may be added to relieve pain. These may include medications that reduce anxiety, promote relaxation or sleep, or reduce muscle tension. Assessment of the type and possible cause of the pain may indicate that some other form of medication is necessary for relief, such as medication for neuroleptic or anginal types of pain.

Transcutaneous stimulation using temperature, pressure, or electrical impulses are useful in addition to or sometimes in the place of medication for relief of acute pain. Application of cold to the painful area results in slight numbing of the area. The sensation of cold is sent as a message to the central nervous system, short circuiting the gate control mechanism for pain. Decrease in local body temperature results in slight vasoconstriction of the area, reducing local circulation as well as limiting the amount of extracellular fluid leaking into the area. Limiting extracellular fluid reduces or prevents swelling. Swelling, through increased local pressure, may increase or even be a cause of pain. It is important to protect the skin when using application of cold to relieve pain. Ice should not be applied directly, rather it should be wrapped in a towel or cloth. Cold should be applied intermittently. A good rule is 20 minutes on—20 minutes off. Continuous application of cold could result in tissue damage as the result of continued vasoconstriction. Clients who use cold or ice for comfort are often reluctant to remove it, because discomfort may recur with rewarming of the area. Therefore, client education is essential in using ice as a method of pain management.

> When using heat or cold therapy to relieve pain, do not use continually or the client will be at risk for tissue injury. Instead, use the hot or cold pack for 20 minutes on, then remove for 20 minutes, then apply for 20 minutes, etc. Carefully assess the skin prior to reapplying.

Use of heat in pain relief is another common choice. Warmth often promotes muscular relaxation and a sense of comfort. Decreasing muscular tension may reduce pain sensations. Vasodilatation occurs locally in the area where heat is applied. This increases circulation, enhancing the removal of cellular debris, toxins, and extracellular fluid from the area of tissue injury. Although heat is not useful in preventing swelling, it is a great aid in reducing swelling that has already occurred. Reduction in swelling may enhance comfort. As with the application of cold, care should be taken to protect the skin where heat is applied. The older client or one with neuropathy is at risk for burns when heat injury is not noticed. Clients with mental status changes or who are sedated should also refrain from using heat for pain relief without supervision, as injury may result. Continuous application of heat is contraindicated for a variety of reasons. The same 20 on—20 off rule used when applying cold is a good idea.

Increased circulation to the area may result in vascular congestion and weeping of extracellular fluid, actually exacerbating swelling. Temperature of any heating device, even a warm water compress, should be carefully checked to prevent burns. Finally, heat should never be applied to an area where there is arterial vascular insufficiency. In this instance, metabolism and oxygen need are increased, putting the client in danger of injury from oxygen deficit.

Benefits of heat and cold therapy:	
Cold	**Hot**
Prevent swelling	Reduce swelling
Reduce swelling	Increase circulation
Sensation of numbness	Promote muscle relaxation
	Decrease muscle spasms

Cutaneous stimulation in the forms of touch, pressure, or massage is another alternative for pain control. Simple touch or pressure applied continuously to one area or superficial massage short circuit the pain sensation gate, sending alternate messages to the central nervous system. These can be useful even when the pain is not superficial. Effleurage, a gentle, rhythmic, superficial stimulation of the skin of the abdomen, is frequently used as one means of pain management during labor. Light massage or superficial stimulation may also reduce muscle tension and anxiety, and promote sleep. Deep massage reduces muscle tension but must be used judiciously when injury is suspected due to the danger of dislodging emboli that may travel throughout the circulatory system.

Transcutaneous electrical nerve stimulation (TENS) can be used to disrupt the pain message to the central nervous system. This requires particular equipment as well as input from a health care practitioner or rigorous client education before use.

Behavioral measures are another group of interventions used for acute pain management in the adult client. The client must be receptive and motivated to use behavioral interventions, and client teaching is necessary for success. Relaxation, visual imagery, hypnosis and self-hypnosis, diversional activity, and music therapy are some behavioral alternatives. Relaxation can be accomplished through breathing exercises, for example in Lamaze childbirth, or through progressive muscular relaxation. These behavioral alternatives promote reduction of anxiety and muscular tension, as well as promoting rest and sleep. Successful use of behavioral techniques enhances the client's perception of being in control of the pain.

Case Study Revisited

During the night, Mr. B. requests more medication than his q 4-6 hours PRN schedule allows. The nurse checks his traction, assessing that the weights are hanging freely and his leg is in good alignment with the rest of his body. However, his pain is described as dull and cramping in his right thigh. Knowing that muscle spasms are a problem with this type of injury, she administers a muscle relaxant. She assists him to a more comfortable position in bed, re-explains how the traction is working, and shows him how to use the radio that is part of the nurse call/television control system. She leaves him quietly listening to the radio. When she looks in 15 minutes later, he is asleep.

CLIENT INVOLVEMENT IN PAIN MANAGEMENT

The adult client with mild acute pain rarely accesses heath care to manage the pain unless the pain interferes with ADLs or is perceived by the client to indicate a problem. It is more common for the health care provider to see a client with moderate to severe acute pain. Medication is the intervention of choice for moderate to severe pain. Transcutaneous or behavioral methods of pain management are rarely used in place of medication in the client with moderate to severe pain. Rather, they are useful as a way to increase the efficacy of pain medication or to reduce the amount of medication necessary for optimal comfort.

Involving the adult client in the planning and implementation of pain management increases the chance that the plan will be successful. This involvement includes client participation in the assessment process, a careful history, and client education in use of the alternatives chosen for pain relief.

The adult client has the ability to learn how to manage pain, but in this population, learning occurs differently than in children. Adults learn information more effectively if it is perceived as immediately useful and believable. The client who is not motivated to be a part of the pain-relief process or who does not believe that the identified options will be successful in relieving pain will learn less effectively. Barriers such as anxiety and discomfort also hinder learning, which inhibit concentration and recall. The client in pain, or one who is accessing the health care system, may suffer from varying degrees of anxiety. With this in mind, client education for pain management should be instituted prior to elective procedures that may result in intraprocedure or postprocedure pain. Measures to reduce anxiety will be effective in increasing retention of what is learned, as well as potentially contributing to pain relief. Some strategies for reducing anxiety include: providing information about procedures, the client's pain and alternatives for pain relief, considering

> An integral part of the education process is to assess for barriers to communication and learning.

physical comfort in the environment where teaching occurs, and providing psychological comforts including privacy and support.

Adult clients learn through a variety of modalities. Spoken instructions or information are useful, but no one is able to retain all of what is told if the information is offered only once. Anxiety or pain reduces retention. Therefore, important information should be repeated, preferably several times. Information should be offered in small, distinct segments for better retention. Directions should be clear and concrete. Having the client verbally restate information or, even better, demonstrate the materiel being learned is an excellent way of assessing the success of the learning process.

Use of other means of communication increase learning. Providing written information as initial or secondary sources of information is helpful. Written material should be in a language that is easily understood by the client, without complicated technical jargon. Assessment of reading skill should be performed: never assume that a client has the ability to read. Pictures, demonstrations, and audio or videotapes are also excellent ways to share information. Including a significant other in teaching sessions may be helpful, as long as it is acceptable to the client and trust and confidentiality are maintained.

> **Never assume that your client is able to read!** This assumption may prevent the client from obtaining important information shared only in a print format.

Case Study Revisited

Before his surgery, Mr. B. is visited by the nurse anesthetist who teaches him to use the PCA (patient-controlled analgesia) pump, which is meant to assist with pain control after surgery. In addition to explaining how and why the PCA works, she has also brought one to demonstrate how to activate the pump to provide a dose of medication on demand. She instructs Mr. B. on how to administer a demand dose and asks him to return the demonstration. She leaves a printed pamphlet describing the PCA, which also has pictures indicating how it is to be used. She also spends some time teaching Mr. B. some controlled breathing and relaxation exercises.

CREATING A PLAN OF CARE

After assessing the pain or potential for pain, creating a plan of care with client involvement includes documentation and sharing of intervention information. The North American Nursing Diagnosis Association (NANDA) classifications[1] are one common method of nursing documentation, identifying and defining client problems. A written plan of care is useful for easily sharing information with the client and with other health care professionals. The written plan of care also streamlines the evaluation process. Setting *realistic* goals for pain relief is very important. In many instances, complete absence of pain is neither realistic nor possible. Verifying client expectations and providing honest information about what he or she can expect will prevent failure.

After assessment, the plan includes identifying measures for pain relief. These include pharmacological as well as nonpharmacological measures, considering availability of resources, and client receptiveness to offered alternatives. Medications that are appropriate for the type, severity, and location of the pain are identified with appropriate dose and route. Careful attention is paid to client allergy and medication use history. Use of a medication that has failed to provide relief for this client in the past is rarely indicated. This would reduce the client's belief in the possibility of relief, as well as potentially reducing client acceptance and adherence with the plan.

Creative combinations of medication along with behavioral and physiological or transcutaneous alternatives increase the potential for success of pain relief. All aspects of the designed plan of care should be used for optimal success. The client should demonstrate understanding that components of the combination approach are not designed to be used individually, rather that all used together constitute the plan for success. Behavioral and physiological measures for comfort are not meant to replace the use of medication, although need for medication may be reduced by adding other types of interventions to the plan of care.

Client acceptance, satisfaction, and adherence to the plan is affected by the client's understanding of the plan, as well as the availability of resources and his or her belief that the plan of care will be successful. Even the most carefully thought out plan of care is worthless if it is not utilized effectively by the client and other health care professionals. When identifying adjunctive methods for pain relief, consider the client's cultural and religious beliefs, which may indicate alternatives or restrict use of some already identified.

One creative way of increasing client participation and facilitating evaluation of the plan of care is through journaling. By encouraging the client to keep a journal of pain experienced and interventions utilized, information becomes available that will assist in modifying the plan. This can be a free-form written journal, a flow sheet, or a timed chart.

Information to include in the journal would be occurrence (time), severity, and location of the pain; precipitating factors; and interventions used. Journaling improves client recall of pain and relief sensations. It is useful in tracking trends for relief and precipitating factors. It presents vital information for evaluation and plan revision. In the case of inpatient treatment with minimal client involvement or when the client is unable to journal, keeping a pain relief flow sheet or chart is a useful alternative. Some clients report the act of keeping a journal is therapeutic in itself; it provides a greater sense of being in control.

Continual assessment of the client's reports of pain as well as ability to accomplish ADLs should be used to evaluate the success of the plan of care. Evaluation includes revision of the plan when optimal relief is not achieved. An important part of client education is to offer and reinforce the idea that initial failure to relieve the pain does not indicate hopelessness. Reassuring the client that multiple medical and nonmedical alternatives exist for pain management and that through continual evaluation and revision an appropriate and useful plan of care will be established. Encourage consistent client feedback in the evaluation process. In cases of difficult pain management, the heath care provider should identify and utilize other resources, such as pain management specialists or clinics and review new literature. It is a realistic goal to strive for optimal pain management for all adult clients with or at risk for episodes of acute pain.

Case Study Resolved

For the first 24 hours after surgery, Mr. B. is quite uncomfortable. Although he is able to use the PCA morphine pump to control pain adequately, he suffers from severe nausea and vomiting. On the second postoperative day, the plan of care is to change his medication to an oral form. The nausea prevents this. His primary nurse knows that nausea and vomiting can be an anesthesia side effect; however, it rarely lasts as long as 24 hours. She also knows that some clients develop nausea and vomiting when using morphine. Although this has not been indicated in Mr. B.'s medication history, she discusses it with the anesthetist, and the medication in the PCA pump is changed to meperidine (Demerol). The nausea resolves, Mr. B. is able to tolerate food and fluids, and on the third postoperative day his pain is well relieved by two Percocet tablets every 6 hours. He uses controlled breathing and relaxation exercises after physical therapy sessions. Mr. B. keeps a flow chart of his pain, the medication used, and what other methods he is using to control his pain. He is discharged home on this very effective regimen on postoperative day 4.

REFERENCE

1. North American Nursing Diagnosis Association. *NANDA Nursing Diagnoses: Definitions and Classification, 1999-2000.* Philadelphia, Pa: Author; 1999.

BIBLIOGRAPHY

Acute Pain Management Clinical Practice Guideline Panel. *Acute Pain Management: Operative or Medical Procedures and Trauma. AHCPR Pub No. 92-0032.* Rockville, Md: Agency for Health Care Policy and Research, US Department of Health and Human Services, Public Health Service; 1992.

McCaffery M, Pasero C. *Pain: Clinical Manual.* 2nd ed. St. Louis, Mo: Mosby; 1999.

MULTIPLE-CHOICE QUESTIONS

1. Signs and symptoms of acute pain include:
   A. Crying, grimacing, elevation in blood pressure and cardiac rate
   B. Flushing, tachycardia, fever
   C. Diaphoresis, pallor, bradycardia
   D. Stoicism, tachypnea, bradycardia

2. Causes of acute pain include:
   A. Trauma
   B. Hypoxia
   C. Bacterial infection
   D. All of the above

3. The process for managing acute pain in correct order include:
   A. Evaluation, intervention, assessment
   B. Assessment, intervention, evaluation, reintervention if necessary
   C. Intervention, evaluation
   D. Assessment, intervention

4. Adjuvant medications are:
   A. Medications that do not require a prescription
   B. Medications given in conjunction with a pain medication to enhance relief
   C. Medications given in place of an ineffective pain medication
   D. Medications given to relieve side effects of a pain medication

5. Cold therapy may be used to relieve pain. When teaching a client to apply cold to an area, it is important to include the following information:
   A. Place ice directly to the painful area
   B. Use cold compresses or ice continually for 24 hours
   C. Do not apply cold to dependent limbs
   D. Apply cold to the area for 20 minutes on, then 20 minutes off; repeat

6. Use of heat to an area to relieve pain is effective because:
   A. Heat allows for increased uptake of opioids in the affected area
   B. Heat promotes muscular relaxation
   C. Heat promotes vasoconstriction, reducing swelling and local edema
   D. Heat promotes systemic vasodilatation

7. In a client education experience, anxiety or pain mediate learning in what way?
   A. They heighten awareness, allowing for increased retention
   B. They lower arousal thresholds, allowing for longer periods of learning
   C. They inhibit attention and reduce retention
   D. They decrease arousal, resulting in resistance to learning

8. A critical part of the plan of care to prevent or relieve pain includes:
   A. Careful assessment and history taking
   B. Formulation of a set of interventions
   C. Documentation of the plan to share with other health care professionals
   D. All of the above

9. Goals for a plan of care to relieve or prevent pain must be:
   A. Realistic and measurable
   B. Idealistic
   C. Attainable through the use of medication
   D. Involved and difficult to enact

10. When initial interventions are not successful to promote pain relief:
    A. It is important to reassure the client that other alternatives are available and to re-evaluate goals
    B. It is important to continue to use those interventions until they work
    C. A medical consult is in order
    D. Acknowledge that it may be impossible to achieve any level of pain relief

MULTIPLE-CHOICE ANSWERS

1. A. An increase in heart rate and elevated blood pressure are the usual manifestations of acute pain. Vital signs and other manifestations, however, may vary. At times, blood pressure may decrease with severe pain.

2. D. All of the above can be causes of acute pain.

3. B. Assessment is critical to planning intervention; intervention must be followed by evaluation, with further intervention utilized as indicated.

4. B. Adjuvant medications enhance the activity of a pain medication or target other symptoms such as anxiety and muscular tension, which may exacerbate pain.

5. D. Intermittent application of cold therapy to the painful area will prevent tissue damage, which could result from vasoconstriction.

6. B. Heat promotes muscular relaxation and comfort. It also promotes local vasodilatation, enhancing the removal of debris, toxins, and extracellular fluid.

7. C. They reduce the client's ability to attend to information, resulting in reduced ability to learn.

8. D. All of the above are critical to the formulation of a good plan of care.

9. A. Goals must be realistic for the client, the setting, the physical circumstances surrounding the pain, and for the health care provider.

10. A. Make sure goals are realistic and attainable, and reassure the client that if one set of interventions is not useful, other interventions targeting the cause or manifestations of the pain are possible.

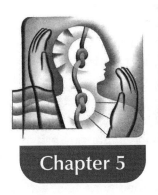

Chapter 5

Pain in the Surgical Client

Case Study

Mrs. O. is a 68-year-old woman who is admitted through the day surgery unit for an elective right modified radical mastectomy for breast cancer. She has been part of a creative preoperative program at the facility, in which she has participated in classes about postoperative pain control, exercise, and postmastectomy care. On the morning of her admission, she is quite anxious about her surgery. Her greatest reported fear is that she will have severe, uncontrolled pain after the surgery. She and her physician have chosen to use PCA after surgery. The PCA routine is reviewed, and the admitting nurse reassures Mrs. O. that other alternatives are certainly available if PCA does not seem to be effective enough.

Pain is an almost universal phenomenon in instances of surgical intervention and trauma. Surgery is an invasive intervention with the intention of treating, controlling, curing, or stabilizing a medical problem. Surgery has many inherent risks, as attested to by the process of informed consent for both surgery and anesthesia. Despite these risks, the primary fear of clients who are about to have surgery is pain: Will it hurt? How will I (the client) deal with it? How can it be treated or prevented? Surgical intervention is an alternative for most client populations, from the very young to the very old. The invasive intervention of surgery is even a choice for clients in special populations who require specific and different assessments and interventions for the resulting pain. It is a primary reason for admission to an acute care facility.

Invasive diagnostic procedures and surgery all carry the threat of pain before, during, and after the procedure. It is the responsibility of the health care team to assess, prevent, and relieve that pain.

Surgery can be emergent in nature, unexpected, or planned. In these cases, pain management is purely postoperative. In other cases, the operative procedure is elective, allowing for a plan of care to prevent or manage pain, as well as client education in utilizing pain management techniques. Although prior preparation would seem to be the preferred alternative, it is a responsibility of the heath care team to attempt to manage pain in either alternative. Surgical intervention is a choice of treatment for countless conditions. It is used to repair traumatic damage in the case of accident or injury, treat congenital anomalies, remove foreign bodies or disease, reduce inflammation as a pain relief alternative, improve function, change appearance, childbirth, or as an exploratory or diagnostic procedure. An operative procedure may be curative, restorative, controlling, or palliative. Considering the reasons for surgery, as well as prior preparation and the personal meaning of the procedure to the client are all important in planning for pain management.

Historically, surgery was done in a hospital environment. The client was admitted to the facility sometimes days before the procedure. The preoperative time was used for assessment, physical preparation, and client education. Recently, changes in technology and reimbursement issues have resulted in changes in where surgery is performed, as well as opportunities for preoperative assessment or client preparation. Now, surgical procedures may be performed in acute care hospitals or inpatient or outpatient units, in freestanding surgicenters, in physicians' or dentists' offices, in clinics and birthing centers. Minor surgical procedures, such as inserting central venous access lines, that were previously done in the hospital may now be done in a long-term care facility or even in the client's own home. When elective surgery is done, even as an inpatient, clients are rarely admitted to the facility days prior to the procedure. Commonly, admission to the surgical facility is on the day of surgery through a day surgery unit. Postoperatively, the client may recover on the day surgery unit and go home that afternoon or evening or be admitted to an inpatient unit. In either case, opportunities for preoperative assessment and preparation for pain management are rare. With increased mobility of clients into and out of facilities pre- and postoperatively, the health care team faces two new challenges: timely and appropriate client education regarding pain management, and telephone triage to manage pain issues outside of the inpatient facility. Client education will be discussed later in this chapter.

Telephone triage is a method of assessment by phone used to evaluate the condition of the client, as well as provide appropriate interventions for presented client problems. It is a therapeutic exchange, involving assessment and treatment that requires the participation of a trained professional who can legally engage in these two activities. It should not be left to an office secretary or answering service.

Triage is a formal procedure, with assessment parameters arranged to identify emergent or life-threatening symptoms and appropriate interventions, which may include activation of emergency services. Assessment criteria are also used to evaluate for less threatening problems. A triage manual should exist for the practice, with written protocols for assessment and interventions. Complete documentation of each triage contact, including assessment, interventions suggested, client response, and resources used, is essential. A system for follow-up evaluation is also a good idea, and it enhances client satisfaction.

Principles of effective triage:
1. Triage is managed by qualified, licensed personnel.
2. Assessment is systematic.
3. A triage manual is used for assessment and intervention; this manual is regularly reviewed.
4. Complete documentation of each triage contact is maintained.
5. A system for follow-up is used.

Triage for the management of postoperative pain and potential complications should be available 24 hours a day, and it is imperative that the client and family are aware of how to seek out assistance from the triage service.

ACUTE PAIN RELATED TO SURGICAL PROCEDURES

Acute pain is pain that lasts for a relatively short duration, usually no more than 3 to 6 months. Clients rarely anticipate that operative pain will last that long. The goals concerning surgical pain include management of pain prior to surgery, prevention of intraoperative pain or sensation, and prevention or relief of postoperative pain during recovery and rehabilitation.

Preoperative pain is a result of disease or injury. Postoperative pain arises from a wide variety of sources and causes. It is important to evaluate and treat the specific types of pain during the pain experience.

Surgical pain management includes:
• Preoperative pain
• Intraoperative pain
• Postoperative pain
• Acute and chronic pain during rehabilitation

Because surgery is invasive, most clients will admit to *incisional pain*, occurring secondary to impaired skin integrity from a scalpel or trocar entry into the body. Incisional pain can be quite severe, because it is cutaneous or peripheral pain. The skin and subcutaneous tissues have a rich supply of nociceptors, which readily transmit the pain message to the central nervous system. It is frequently described as cutting, searing, burning, sharp pain. It can be more severe in certain areas of the body. For example, incisional pain is often quite severe in the axillary area following an axillary node dissection. Incisional pain can also occur in response to stretching or pulling of skin tissues during surgery and in response to irritation from surgical prep solutions such as providine iodine (Betadine, Perdue-Frederick, Norwalk, Conn) or tape placed against the skin after surgery. Anxiety can also impact incisional pain, such as when a client manifests fear of disfigurement. The incision is usually covered with dressings immediately after surgery, and clients are often left to imagine what it looks like. With a fear of disfigurement, the incision and resultant scar can become an important source of anxiety, reinforcing or exacerbating the incisional pain. Allowing clients to view the incisional area, as well as careful client teaching regarding the mode of closure (stitches, staples, Steristrips), may help reduce anxiety in these situations, leading to improved pain control.

Somatic and *visceral* types of pain are commonly associated with surgical intervention. They are a result of surgical manipulation or removal of target organs for treatment purposes, as well as pressure from manipulation of surrounding tissues. These types of pain may also be related to swelling, fluid accumulation, or hematoma formation around the surgical area. Somatic pain arises in muscles, bone joints, ligaments, or fascia. It is structural pain and may occur at rest or with movement. Visceral pain is organ pain. It arises in the abdominal, pelvic, thoracic, or cranial cavities. Both are the result of stimulation of deeper nociceptors. Visceral pain can be diffuse and poorly localized; somatic pain is more specifically localized. Both may be constant or intermittent in nature. Client descriptions vary from sharp and severe to dull and achy. This type of pain is rarely described as burning or searing. It is the "expected" type of pain experienced after surgery or childbirth. Successful relief measures include a variety of pharmacological and nonpharmacological alternatives. Anxiety can also be a significant component in this type of pain, resulting in increased muscular tension with an accompanying increase in levels of pain.

Neuropathic pain is another type of pain frequently associated with surgery. It occurs because of surgical disruption or destruction of nerve fibers, either superficially on incision or deeper within the body. It can also be related to pressure or inflammation as irritants to the nerves in the surgical area. A client's description of neuropathic pain is usually characteristic—there is a hot, burning, or searing quality. Neuropathic pain is frequently resistant to common interventions for postsurgical pain and requires specific interventions.

Many clients will complain about pain or aches that seem unrelated to the surgical procedure. Some common complaints include a sore throat, lower back pain, and limb or joint pain. Although it is important to assess each client who offers these complaints individually for signs of infection or injury, quite often these symptoms are related to the process of surgery. A sore throat is often related to intubation during anesthesia. A client undergoing a procedure including general anesthesia will often have an endotracheal tube placed to facilitate the delivery of anesthetic gases and oxygen, and to protect from aspiration. The tube is usually placed after the client has entered an anesthetic sleep, and unless intubation and ventilation are required after the surgery, the tube is removed in the operating room or postanesthesia care unit before the client is aware of it. The irritation of the tube against the back of the pharynx may leave the client with a sore throat.

Back and limb pains are often the result of positioning during surgery. The operating table is a relatively hard, rigid surface with minimal padding. This is for functional and safety reasons. After anesthesia has been administered, the client is positioned to allow the surgeon optimal access to the surgical area. Despite the fact that the client's body is padded and handled safely, these positions may cause muscle soreness postoperatively because of the long period of time the client has been maintained in possibly an awkward position on a hard surface. Clients who have orthopedic surgery, especially joint surgery, may complain of pain as a result of manipulation to position or seat the joint as part of the surgical procedure. Back or shoulder pain may also be related to insufflation of the abdominal cavity with gas

> Positioning during a surgical procedure can sometimes lead to inadvertent pain or injury. Mr. W. complained of pain and a 2-inch circular bruise on his left thigh. He was recovering from replacement of his right hip. The bruise was a result of one of the surgical team leaning his elbow against Mr. W.'s left thigh to gain leverage during this difficult orthopedic surgery.

during abdominal or pelvic arthroscopic surgery. Although a major portion of the gas is removed by suction prior to final closure, some free gas remains in the abdominal cavity.

Once the client sits or stands upright, the gas floats upward, exerting pressure on the diaphragm and creating characteristic shoulder and upper back pain. This is no cause for alarm. The client's body will safely absorb the gas in a short period of time, usually over the next 24 hours. Careful explanation about the reasons for these types of pain, as well as the commonality of their occurrence, may enhance other interventions for the pain.

After surgery, the client may admit to pain that does not appear to be directly related to the surgical procedure or to the processes described above. This pain is often related to the consequences of decreased mobility. Abdominal pain and cramping, especially of the lower abdomen, is a frequent complaint. It may occur in a client who has had abdominal or pelvic surgery or in one who has had surgery on a completely separate part of the body. The client who complains of this type of pain after abdominal or pelvic surgery is most likely suffering from decreased intestinal motility. Peristalsis tends to slow or completely stop when the intestines have been handled or pushed out of the operative field. Assess for bowel sounds in all four quadrants, as well as for flatus and bowel activity since the surgery. In the absence of bowel sounds, the client should remain NPO. Decreased intestinal motility can also occur as the result of physical mobility, for example in the case of a client who has had orthopedic surgery followed by several days of complete bedrest. It can also be related to opioid use, resulting in retention of gas and constipation. This type of abdominal pain is not responsive to treatment with narcotics; in fact, narcotics may further slow intestinal motility and exacerbate the pain. An increase in the client's level of activity, with frequent ambulating, will enhance intestinal motility. Use of a cathartic suppository may also be considered.

Leg or calf pain is another type of pain that occurs after surgery, especially when the client has been immobilized for a prolonged period. This pain may indicate a deep vein thrombosis (DVT), a potentially dangerous complication of immobility. The primary danger of DVT is embolization. The client who experiences leg or calf pain must be promptly assessed for accompanying signs of redness, swelling, and warmth to the area, as well as tenderness and fever. The client should immediately be placed on complete bedrest, and massage to the limb must be avoided. Application of moist heat may relieve the pain. With the diagnosis of DVT, anticoagulant therapy will be instituted.

Inflammation is a protective mechanism used by the body in a variety of circumstances to prevent injury to tissues and to remove foreign bodies or debris. It is primarily mediated by the immune system. Inflammation results in increased circulation to the affected area, with movement of fluid across vessel and cellular barriers. The consequences of an inflammatory reaction include redness (from increased circulation), swelling, heat, or increased metabolic activity and pain. Inflammation can be seen in the client as a normal response in the operative area or as a response to infection or allergy. It is a significant source of pain. The goal of maintaining comfort in the postoperative client has two components: to prevent inflammation and to reduce the inflammatory response, relieving the discomfort it causes. If the surgical area is peripheral, such as an arm or leg, maintaining the limb elevated above the level of the client's heart will prevent some swelling. Assessment for signs and symptoms of infection or hematoma formation allow for early treatment to prevent extensive inflammation. Hematoma formation is important because the old blood that accumulates in the area is an excellent source for infection, as well as a signal to the body for activity to commence to remove the debris. For this reason, surgical clients often have drains placed at the operative area. Heat and cold therapy are both used to help resolve inflammation and enhance comfort. Including anti-inflammatory medication in the pain relief regimen will also add to comfort.

Case Study Revisited

Mrs. O. is admitted to the inpatient surgical unit from the PACU at 1:15 pm. The PACU nurse reports that Mrs. O. has ranked her pain as 3 out of 10 and that she is using the PCA appropriately. At change of shift, Mrs. O. tells the nurse that her pain is "around a 6"; she is diaphoretic and her pulse and blood pressure are elevated. The PCA pump report documents that Mrs. O. has received all of the medication the program allows, so the nurse gets an order from anesthesia for a bolus and an increase in the programmed doses. Within 1 hour, Mrs. O. states she is pain-free and her vital signs have returned to baseline.

At 6:00 pm, Mrs. O. refuses her meal, stating that she is quite nauseated. Despite treatment with prochlorperazine (Compazine, SmithKline Beecham, Research Triangle Park, NC) and ondansetron (Zofran, Glaxo Wellcome, Research Triangle Park, NC), Mrs. O. vomits twice and is very uncomfortable with the nausea. The anesthesiologist elects to discontinue using the morphine on the PCA pump and orders PCA meperidine (Demerol) instead. Mrs. O.'s nausea resolves and her pain is well-controlled using the meperidine.

CHRONIC PAIN IN THE POSTOPERATIVE PERIOD

Chronic pain has a longer duration than acute pain, lasting more than 6 months. It may be constant or intermittent. Chronic pain presents the challenge to the client of maintaining life in the face of pain. It is sometimes accompanied by decreases in mobility, ability for self-care, depression, and role changes. There are two types of chronic pain that are important to consider in the client who has had surgery: (1) pain as a result of the surgery, trauma, or illness; (2) pain that is not related to the surgery but must be managed during the immediate postoperative period. Chronic pain related to the problem that instigated surgery may be expected or unexpected. In some circumstances, it is not reasonable to believe that a client can become pain-free. In other instances, chronic pain occurs because rehabilitation and resumption of baseline levels of activity take longer than 3 to 6 months. Clients who have had aggressive orthopedic, cardiac, or gastrointestinal surgery often spend many months in the rehabilitation process. Chronic postoperative pain may also have a neuropathic element as the result of disruption or destruction of nervous tissue. Phantom pain, which occurs after amputation, is one good example. Chronic pain is often the reason for an elective surgery. Management of chronic postoperative pain is similar to that of other types of chronic pain. It includes establishing realistic goals with the client, frequent evaluation of the plan of care, and a commitment to managing this type of pain, which interferes with the client's return to baseline comfort.

Chronic pain that is unrelated to the surgical procedure is a second challenge to the health care team. Many clients, especially the elderly, undergo elective or emergent surgeries with comorbidities, which cause chronic pain. In addition to addressing surgical pain, assessment of baseline chronic pain and usual pain relief measures are necessary. In the case of osteoarthritis or other types of chronic pain, salicylates or NSAIDs may be the treatment of choice for the client. Medications in both of these classes can cause blood dyscrasias or clotting difficulties. Not only may clients be directed to discontinue use of these medications up to 2 weeks prior to elective surgery, but their use in the period directly after surgery may be limited as well. Acetaminophen is one alternative medication to replace these. In addition to medications, alternate interventions for relief should also be considered, including heat or cold therapy, exercise, and positioning as appropriate. Successful management of pre-existing chronic pain during the surgical period will contribute to a positive client outcome.

Case Study Revisited

Postoperative orders include frequent ambulation on the first postoperative day. Mrs. O. seems reluctant to walk, even with the assistance of a nursing student. During her assessment of the client, the student finds out that Mrs. O. has osteoarthritis in both knees, which is quite painful. Her usual pain relief medication for this is aspirin, but she states she was told by her surgeon to discontinue use of aspirin for at least a week before the surgery. After a call to the doctor, the nurse brings Mrs. O. some ibuprofen for arthritis pain and inflammation. This medication provides good relief and by afternoon, Mrs. O. is ambulating independently.

PAIN MANAGEMENT ALTERNATIVES

A wide variety of alternatives for pain management for the client with surgical pain exists, from medication of multiple types and dosage routes to traditional and nontraditional alternative therapies. Medications are very often prescribed for the surgical client. Pain management during the intraoperative period may be accomplished through the use of general or regional anesthesia, or with conscious sedation. Conscious sedation is a practice in which the client enters a state of twilight sleep but remains arousable and aware of his surroundings. An opioid for pain reduction and a medication that will cause amnesia during the conscious sedation period are usually included. The importance of conscious sedation during surgical or other invasive procedures is that pain is controlled and/or forgotten, but the client is able to cooperate during the procedure as well as maintain his or her own airway. Conscious sedation carries potentials for danger, including respiratory depression, oxygen desaturation, risk for aspiration, and injury. The client must be comprehensively monitored through the sedation period and until recovery is complete.

Use of medication as intervention for postoperative pain is extremely common. According to the AHCPR's clinical guidelines for acute pain management,[1] medication therapy should be a stepped approach. Mild to moderate surgical pain should be treated initially with NSAID therapy (see Table 3-1). These drugs alone can frequently control pain well. Around-the-clock dosage every 4 to 6 hours is often more successful than administering them on an as-needed (PRN) basis. When the client waits until pain is significant to request or take pain medication, either NSAIDs or opioids, control of the pain can become difficult. Frequent assessment and evaluation of pain relief is necessary. Adjuvant methods of pain control can be added to the NSAID therapy. In the event that pain is not well controlled by NSAID therapy or pain is more severe, opioids can be introduced (see Table 3-2).

Opioids can be used in addition to NSAIDs but not necessarily as a replacement. Postoperative dose scheduling should be around the clock and not PRN for at least the first 36 hours after surgery. At this time, further assessment will dictate changes in scheduling or medication. Opioids can be administered through a variety of routes. In acute care facilities, when the client has established intravenous access, an IV route is chosen. The benefits are rapid delivery of medication to the circulatory system and minimal invasiveness. Drawbacks include rapid metabolism and shorter optimum serum medication levels. So the client experiences rapid, but short-term, relief. One excellent choice for many clients who are receiving IV medication for postoperative pain is the patient-controlled analgesia (PCA) pump.

A PCA pump usually connotes IV drug administration; however, intramuscular, subcutaneous, or epidural routes have been used with the PCA pump as well. The client who uses a PCA pump must be able to follow directions, be willing to monitor and control his or her own pain, and be motivated to take control. Ideally, client education about using the pump appropriately should occur in the preoperative period. Postoperatively, pain or medication may interfere with the learning process; however, if preoperative education is not possible, it should not remove PCA as a valuable option.

PCA uses a programmable pump. The client is usually given an initial loading dose and can then request a determined dose of pain medication on demand. Demand usually involves pushing a small request button. The dose is practitioner-determined, as well as the minimum interval allowable between doses and the maximum amount of medication allowed over a set period. Two alternatives are available: (1) the client receives a basal rate of medication, a continuous IV amount in addition to the client-demanded doses; (2) only intermittent doses demanded by the client are administered. This is a safe alternative to intermittent injections of pain medication. Drawbacks to PCA use include misunderstandings on the part of the client, physical or mental inability to use the pump, poor education or preparation for PCA as a pain-relief method, poor IV access, or reluctance on the part of the client to self-medicate for pain.

One of the safety measures of a PCA pump is that as the client becomes sedated from the medication, he or she does not push the demand button. For example, the surgical client's family complained that the client was impossible to arouse. The nurse assessed him to be quite sedated, with a depressed respiratory rate. The client was given a dose of naloxone (Narcan), reversing the activity of the narcotics from the PCA pump. While investigating the incident, it was discovered that the client's wife had listened to the client education about use of the PCA pump. She was aware that her husband could receive a dose of medication through the pump every 8 minutes *if he needed it*. While he slept, she continued to push the PCA pump button every 8 minutes, short circuiting that safety mechanism. It is important to remind clients and their families that PCA pumps should be client-controlled!

Medications commonly used in a PCA pump are morphine and meperidine (Demerol). Since these medications may cause uncomfortable side effects, including nausea and itching, care should be taken to assess for and rapidly treat these problems. In the event of side effects that become a barrier to effective use of the PCA, an alternative medication or administration system should be considered.

Other routes of administration for postoperative pain medication include sublingual or transbuccal, rectal, intramuscular, subcutaneous, or epidural. Transcutaneous administration of postoperative medications is usually not an option because it takes 24 to 48 hours to establish effective serum drug levels, and medication is difficult to titrate using this route.

For the client with mild to moderate pain, the oral route of administration is preferable. It is safe, easy, and economical. In the case of severe pain, oral use of opioids is one possibility; however, IV or epidural administration may provide greater efficacy. Changes in technology, which have made pumps smaller, cheaper, and easy to use have made IV and epidural administration possible outside of the acute care facility. In many parts of the country, these routes of administration of medication for severe pain are even used in the client's own home with support from visiting nurses or ambulatory clinics.

NONPHARMACOLOGICAL CHOICES FOR POSTOPERATIVE PAIN MANAGEMENT

Pain management through nonpharmacological choices is important for the surgical client to use in addition to medications, as well as instead of medications. Choice of nonpharmacological methods should take into account the severity and reasons for the client's pain, as well as the client's motivation to utilize them. These methods are bound to fail if the client does not believe they will be effective or does not wish to use them. In assessing the client and planning for interventions, cognitive ability and awareness, cultural biases, and levels of mobility should be considered. A variety of cognitive approaches are available including relaxation, guided imagery, music therapy, distraction, and hypnosis or self-hypnosis. Ways to reduce anxiety and accompanying muscular tension will be useful. Physical methods of relief including light cutaneous stimulation, deep massage, heat and cold therapies, and exercise are also alternatives. All of these are described at length in other areas of this text. Careful choice of client education formats, including written, verbal, pictures, and video, can reinforce ways to use nonpharmacological methods.

In conclusion, comprehensive assessment and planning are necessary to manage a client's postoperative pain. Each client is seen as an individual with differing causes, responses to, and meanings for pain. It is an important goal for the health care team to proactively prevent severe pain in the postoperative period. Interventions can be more successful if the client has been included in goal setting and has received education about intervention methods. The most beneficial time to do this education is preoperatively, when possible, because pain, anxiety, and medications used postoperatively may be barriers to learning. These factors do no preclude or prevent learning but must be considered when client education occurs after surgery, as all surgical procedures are not elective and preoperative education may be impossible in many cases.

Case Study Resolved

On the second postoperative day, when her oral intake is good, Mrs. O.'s PCA is discontinued and she is started on an oral codeine and acetaminophen tablet. Although she gets good relief, Mrs. O. complains that this medication leaves her feeling light-headed and "spacey." She would prefer not to use it. Since the ibuprofen has relieved her arthritic pain so well, she is maintained on around-the-clock ibuprofen with good relief of the surgical pain as well. She is discharged to home on the fourth postoperative day using this regimen with excellent pain control.

REFERENCE

1. Acute Pain Management Clinical Practice Guideline Panel. *Acute Pain Management: Operative or Medical Procedures and Trauma. AHCPR Pub No. 92-0032.* Rockville, Md: Agency for Health Care Policy and Research, US Department of Health and Human Services, Public Health Service; 1992.

BIBLIOGRAPHY

American Academy of Ambulatory Care Nursing. *Ambulatory Care Nursing Administration and Practice Standards.* Pitman, NJ: Anthony J. Jannetti, Inc; 2000.

American Academy of Ambulatory Care Nursing. *Telephone Nursing Practice Administration and Practice Standards.* Pitman, NJ: Anthony J. Jannetti, Inc; 1997.

Edwards B. Seeing is believing—picture building: a key component of telephone triage. *J Clin Nurs.* 1998;7(1):51-57.

Fairchild S. *Perioperative Nursing: Principles and Practice.* 2nd ed. Boston, Mass: Little, Brown, & Co; 1996.

Girard N. Clients having surgery: promoting positive outcomes. In: Black JK, Hawks JH, Keene AM, eds. *Medical-Surgical Nursing: Clinical Management for Positive Outcomes.* 6th ed. Philadelphia, Pa: WB Saunders; 2001:273-313.

McCaffery M, Pasero C. *Pain: Clinical Manual.* 2nd ed. St. Louis, Mo: Mosby; 1999.

Wheeler SQ, Windt J. *Telephone Triage: Theory, Practice, and Protocol Development.* Albany, NY: Delmar; 1993.

MULTIPLE-CHOICE QUESTIONS

1. Assessment and consideration for pain management following surgery is best begun:

    A. In the postanesthesia care unit

    B. Once the client returns to the surgical unit

    C. Only by a specially trained anesthesiologist

    D. At the same time as other preoperative assessments are instituted

2. Types of pain that are important to consider in the postoperative client when providing pain-relief interventions include:

    A. Acute pain

    B. Chronic pain

    C. Pain unrelated to the surgical intervention

    D. All of the above

3. Mrs. Smith is 36 hours postop following an abdominal hysterectomy. She describes abdominal pain as 7 on a scale of 10. It is cramping in nature and intermittent. Her bowel sounds are hypoactive and she denies passing flatus. The best intervention would be:

    A. Morphine sulfate 10 mg as ordered by MD

    B. Two Percocet tablets, PO as ordered by MD

    C. Ambulation at least twice per shift

    D. No intervention is necessary at this time

4. Incisional pain refers to:

    A. Mild pain experienced 6 to 8 months after surgery

    B. Sharp pain related to damaged nociceptors in the skin and subcutaneous tissues

    C. An allergic response to suture materials

    D. Insignificant, because it is only the result of anxiety

5. Clients complaining of back or limb pain after surgery are:

    A. Manipulating the nursing staff to get more narcotics

    B. Suffering from a phenomenon known as phantom pain

    C. Responding to the result of positioning during surgery

    D. Exhibiting signs of postoperative hemorrhage

6. Back or shoulder pain is frequently reported by clients who have undergone laproscopic surgery of the abdomen or pelvis. This is the result of:

    A. Postoperative anxiety

    B. Placement of an nasogastric tube

    C. Incisional pain

    D. Trapped gas in the abdominal cavity

7. Mr. Allen is recovering from hip replacement surgery. Three days after surgery on his left hip, he complains of right calf pain. The right calf is red, warm, and tender to touch. An appropriate nursing intervention would be:

   A. To immediately place the client on bedrest with the right leg elevated

   B. To treat the right calf with gentle massage

   C. To apply ice to the right calf

   D. To increase ambulation

8. A 78-year-old woman is treated surgically for intestinal blockage. After surgery, ambulation is a priority to reduce complications related to immobility. Prior to her surgery, this client suffered from osteoarthritic pain of both hips and knees, which she treated with aspirin. An appropriate nursing intervention postoperatively would be:

   A. Use of warm, moist heat to the joints before and after ambulation

   B. Reinstituting aspirin therapy

   C. No intervention is necessary, as postoperative narcotics will manage that pain

   D. Vigorous massage to the lower extremities

9. To gain a postoperative client's cooperation in ambulating, coughing, and deep breathing, and turning, which is the most important intervention for the nurse to perform?

   A. Administer analgesics as ordered to ensure the client is relatively comfortable

   B. Be sure that the client understands the rationale for these activities

   C. Warn the client that life-threatening complications may arise if he or she is not cooperative

   D. Praise the client for completed activities

MULTIPLE-CHOICE ANSWERS

1. D
2. D
3. C
4. B
5. C
6. D
7. A
8. A
9. A

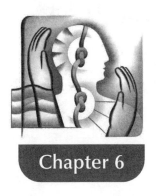

Chapter 6

Pain in the Adult With Cancer

Case Study

J.T. is a 50-year-old client with a 3-year history of lung cancer with metastasis to the bone. For several months she has been experiencing pain that until recently has been well controlled with morphine sulfate sustained release (MSSR) (eg, MS Contin) 15 mg by mouth every 12 hours and occasional morphine sulfate immediate release (MSIR) 10 mg.

Two days ago, J.T. began to have more frequent pain in her right shoulder, which she rated a 7 on a scale of 0 to 10. She took six doses of MSIR 10 mg with good effect. The home health nurse suggested that she contact J.T.'s physician to request an increase in her MSSR to provide better pain control. The doctor orders an increase in J.T.'s MSSR to 30 mg every 12 hours and instructs the client to contact him if the pain continues or gets worse.

One day after increasing her MSSR to 30 mg every 12 hours, J.T. rates her pain as 2 at rest. But the following day, J.T.'s pain rating increases to a 10 despite the increase in MSSR and increased use of MSIR. Today's assessment of pain indicates that the pain in J.T.'s shoulder is now associated with painful sensations shooting down to her thumb and index finger. The nurse recognizes that J.T.'s pain is out of control, that it is likely neuropathic, and that J.T. needs aggressive treatment to control her pain. The nurse instructs J.T. to take a dose of MSIR, and she contacts the physician to arrange immediate treatment. Arrangements are made to transport J.T. by ambulance to the hospital for admission to the inpatient oncology unit with a diagnosis of pain related to metastatic lung cancer.

THE PROBLEM OF CANCER PAIN

Surveys indicate that pain is experienced by approximately one-third of individuals treated for cancer and more than two-thirds with advanced cancer.[1] It is estimated that in

Table 6-1

Barriers to Cancer Pain Management

Problems Related to Health Care Professionals

Inadequate knowledge of pain management
Poor assessment of pain
Concern about regulation of controlled substances
Concern about clients becoming tolerant to analgesics

Problems Related to Clients

Reluctance to report pain
• Concern about distracting physicians from treatment of underlying disease
• Fear that pain means disease is worse
• Concern about not being a "good" patient
Reluctance to take pain medications
• Fear of addiction or of being thought of as an addict
• Worries about unmanageable side effects
• Concern about becoming intolerant to pain medications

Problems Related to the Health Care System

Low priority given to cancer pain treatment
Inadequate reimbursement
The most appropriate treatment is too costly for clients and families
Restrictive regulation of controlled substances
Availability of treatment or access to it

Source: Management of Cancer Pain Guideline Panel. *Managing Cancer Pain Clinical Practice Guideline. AHCPR Pub No. 94-0595.* Rockville, Md: Agency for Health Care Policy and Research, Public Health Service, US Department of Health and Human Services; 1994.

almost all (98% and 99%) cases, clients could have their pain adequately relieved using available knowledge and tools. Despite the existence of effective treatment regimens and the availability of guidelines to facilitate treatment, surveys suggest that more than 40% to 50% of clients in routine practice settings fail to achieve adequate pain relief.

Multiple barriers to effective management of cancer pain have been identified (Table 6-1). Inadequate knowledge of pain management on the part of health care professionals has been cited as a key barrier. The purpose of this book is to educate current and future health care providers about clinical problems in the management of pain that they may not encounter in traditional curricula. Hopefully it will enlighten providers in such a way that improvements in the management of cancer pain occur and more relief is achieved.

Pharmacological management of cancer pain following the World Health Organization analgesic ladder is well-described in Chapter 3 of this text. The purpose of this chapter is to describe the problem of cancer pain characterized by an increase in intensity over hours to days.

TYPES OF CANCER PAIN

Pain related to cancer can be classified according to its etiology, its origin and character, and its duration. There are three broad etiologies of cancer pain:

1. Pain associated with a tumor
2. Pain associated with cancer therapy
3. Pain unrelated to the cancer or its treatment

Pain associated with a tumor is responsible for the majority of pain related to cancer. An example of this type of pain would be abdominal pain related to a colorectal tumor obstructing the large colon. Nerve damage secondary to chemotherapy resulting in peripheral neuropathy is an example of pain related to cancer therapy. Pain related to appendicitis is an example of pain unrelated to cancer or the treatment.

Cancer pain can also be classified according to its origin and character. Nociceptive pain refers to pain that is directly related to tumor infiltration of either somatic (eg, joint, muscle, bone) or visceral (eg, gastrointestinal tract) structures. Somatic pain is characterized as well-localized, deep, dull, or achy. The underlying cause is usually an inflammatory process. Bone metastasis, incisional pain, and wound pain are examples of somatic pain. Visceral pain originating from gastrointestinal tract structure is characterized as poorly localized, vague pressure that is often constricting or cramping. Visceral pain is often present in clients with advanced colon or ovarian cancers secondary to stretching of the mesentery and abdominal organs.

Neuropathic pain applies to a variety of pain syndromes characterized by aberrant or somatosensory processes that originate in the peripheral or central nervous system. It is described as sharp, burning, shooting, shocklike, or electric. Sources of neuropathic pain involve tumor invasion of nerves, post-herpetic neuralgia, chemical damage to nerves from chemotherapy, surgical interruption of nerves, or spinal nerve root compression.

Cancer pain is also classified in terms of duration, with acute pain generally being defined as lasting less than 1 to 3 months and chronic pain lasting longer than 3 to 6 months. Pain related to an unresectable or recurrent tumor is generally chronic in duration.

Pain that occurs intermittently in clients with chronic cancer pain is described as *episodic*. Episodic pain can be categorized in three distinct ways: incident pain, end-of-dose pain, and breakthrough pain. *Incident pain* is related to a particular activity or experience, such as getting out of bed or reacting to an emotional stimuli such as fear. *End-of-dose pain* occurs when the effect of a long-acting analgesic is not sustained over an expected duration. *Breakthrough pain* is a transitory episode of pain that is rapid in onset and usually of short duration (< 30 minutes). Breakthrough pain occurs despite adequate titration of long-acting opioids or continuous intravenous (IV) opioid drips.

Chronic cancer pain is ideally treated with around-the-clock medication to maintain a consistent blood level of analgesic, with the goal of preventing episodes of pain. To achieve a consistent level of analgesic, clients with chronic cancer pain who are able to swallow oral medications are often treated with long-acting opioids such as morphine sulfate sustained release (MS Contin, Oramorph, Purdue-Frederick, Norwalk, Conn) or sustained-release oxycodone (Oxycontin SR). If a client is not able to safely swallow a long-acting oral preparation, he or she may need to receive a continuous opioid drip given intravenously or subcutaneously. Long-acting preparations must not be crushed or broken.

Treatment of episodic pain in the individual with chronic cancer pain requires short-acting analgesics that have a rapid onset. Morphine sulfate immediate release (MSIR) given orally or intravenously is the preferred method. Morphine injections are avoided because they cause pain and because variations in absorption make it difficult to titrate medication to achieve a steady state of analgesia. Incident pain, such as pain related to movement, may be treated prophylactically prior to an event (eg, getting out of bed). End-of-dose pain generally requires an increase in around-the-clock or long-acting opioids.

In contrast to end-of-dose pain, breakthrough pain occurs despite adequate round-the-clock levels of analgesia. Because the level of analgesia is considered adequate, an increase in long-acting or continuous opioids is not the treatment of choice for true breakthrough pain. However, it is not uncommon for health care providers to increase doses of long-acting opioids to "cover" or prevent breakthrough pain. An increase in the long-acting opioid for breakthrough pain is not ideal because it can lead to an overintensification of side effects and oversedation. Some health care providers believe that the preferred treatment for breakthrough pain is to give a fast-acting opioid with rapid clearance. Though oral MSIR is generally used for this purpose, it is not the ideal drug for breakthrough pain because it may take more than 30 minutes to take effect, with a peak effect in 40 to 60 minutes. Breakthrough pain typically lasts less than 30 minutes, and the onset of MSIR may not be fast enough to treat breakthrough pain adequately. A faster acting opioid such as fentanyl may be more appropriate for breakthrough pain, but more studies are needed to identify the appropriate oral dose.

CHRONIC CANCER PAIN

The intensity of chronic cancer pain varies from mild or moderate to severe or excruciating. Most clients describe their cancer pain as mild to moderate. If an increase in the intensity of chronic cancer pain occurs, prompt medical attention is warranted to fully assess the pain and determine its origin. Increased pain often represents progression of cancer, particularly in advanced disease. However, new pain in a person with cancer may also be a sign of infection, fracture, or a neurological problem.

> Increase in pain often represents progression of the cancer, particularly in advanced disease. However, new pain in a person with cancer may also be a sign of infection, fracture, or a neurological problem, which may be reversible.

It is essential that client reports of a "new" pain be thoroughly explored to ensure that a reversible complication (such as spinal cord compression) is not overlooked. Reports of pain, especially of increased severity, or at a new location must not automatically be attributed to a pre-existent cause or to opioid tolerance. Although much has been written about opioid tolerance, tolerance is seldom the cause of increased cancer pain.

Knowledge of relationships that certain cancers have with pain patterns and patterns of metastasis helps determine the etiology of new pain. Patterns of metastasis help determine the etiology of new pain. Multiple myeloma and cancers of the breast, prostate, and lung account for the majority of cancers with bone metastasis that frequently is characterized by pain. Pain from bone is caused by direct tumor involvement of bone with activation of nociceptors or from compression of adjacent nerves, vascular structures, and soft tissue. With multiple sites involved, clients with bone metastasis commonly have multiple areas of pain. Complications of bone metastasis, such as pathological fractures or spinal cord compression, can lead to additional sources for pain and morbidity. Spinal cord or epidural compression commonly occurs with cancers of the breast, prostate, lung, kidney; multiple myeloma; or malignant melanoma.

Plexopathies caused by an infiltration of nerves by the tumor or compression of nerves by fibrosis are another source of cancer-related pain. Cervical plexopathy is commonly related to primary head and neck cancers with local metastasis. Brachial plexopathy is commonly related to cancers of the breast, lung, and lymphoma, but it can also occur as metastasis from a more distant tumor. Lumbosacral plexopathy can occur by direct spread from colorectal, endometrial, or renal cancers; sarcomas; or lymphomas. Peripheral neuropathy related to cancer pain can occur when peripheral nerves are infiltrated by tumor or constricted by fibrosis. Multiple myeloma causes a peripheral neuropathy in about 15% of clients. Peripheral nerves can also be damaged by neurotoxic chemotherapy such as vincristine, cisplatin, and paclitaxel (Taxol). Peripheral nerve damage can also occur after cutaneous incisions and retraction of tissues during surgery.

Neuralgia resulting from infection or reactivation of varicella-zoster virus is another cause of pain related to cancer. This neuralgia can cause both acute and chronic pain and commonly affects thoracic and cranial dermatomes.

Case Study Revisited

The escalation of J.T.'s pain is found to be related to metastasis of her lung cancer to the brachial plexus. The diagnosis of this new pain source is facilitated by J.T.'s description that the pain feels like a shooting, electric sensation in her thumb and index finger that begins in the right shoulder. Knowledge that this pain likely represents the neuropathic pain characteristic of brachial plexopathy and that the relationship of brachial plexopathy with lung cancer prompts the physician to validate the diagnosis by computed tomography.

TREATMENT OF NEUROPATHIC PAIN

Neuropathic pain is considered one of the most difficult types of pain to control. Although it is less responsive to opioids than nociceptive pain, opioids are the first line of treatment, with morphine sulfate the drug of choice. Because neuropathic pain is less responsive to opioids, higher doses are generally required for its relief and control.

Opioids have a wide range of effect and their effect is dependent on the individual's partic-

> Neuropathic pain is described as sharp, burning, shooting, shock-like, or electric.

ular response to the drug. Thus, one person's pain might respond well to a low dose of opioid, which may provide little if any effect for another's pain. When using opioids without a ceiling dose, the amount of the drug that the person requires for relief and control of pain is not as important as is the individual's ability to tolerate side effects. Increases in opioids (without a ceiling dose) for uncontrolled cancer pain are acceptable as long as there is a balance between the medication's beneficial effect and its adverse effects.

Although respiratory depression is a potential risk when opioid doses are increased, it has not been found to be a common problem for individuals who have been receiving opioids for a long period of time or for clients with excruciating pain. Sedation as a side effect tends to be a more common reason for limiting opioids in clients with chronic cancer. Nausea can be another dose-limiting factor for use of opioids. Intermittent doses of antiemetics can often be given to prevent or treat nausea or vomiting related to opioids. Nausea related to narcotics also can be temporary, subsiding within a few days of opioid

Table 6-2

Adjuvant Analgesics for Neuropathic Cancer Pain

Class	Generic Name	Trade Name
Antidepressants		
Tricyclic antidepressants	Amitriptyline	Elavil
	Desipramine	Norpramin
	Doxepin	Sinequan
	Imipramine	Tofranil
	Nortriptyline	Pamelor
Nontricyclic antidepressants	Trazodone	Desyrel
	Maprotiline	Ludiomil
	Fluoxetine	Prozac
	Paroxetine	Paxil
Anticonvulsants	Carbamazepine	Tegretol
	Phenytoin	Dilantin
	Valproate	Depakote
	Clonazepam	Klonopin
	Gabapentin	Neurontin
Local anesthetics/antiarrhythmics	Lidocaine	Xylocaine
	Mexiletine	Mexitil
	Tocainide	Tonocard
Corticosteroids	Dexamethasone	Decadron
	Prednisone	Deltasone
Miscellaneous	Baclofen	Lioresal
	Clonidine	Catapres
	Capsaicin cream	Capzasin P

increases. However, nausea and vomiting, as well as other side effects, may be unmanageable when opioid doses are increased. If a client has unmanageable side effects on a high dose of one opioid, the recommendation is to change to a different opioid at 50% of the equianalgesic amount of the first opioid to assess for tolerance. If severe opioid toxicity occurs, the recommendation is to switch to a dose even lower than 50% of the first equianalgesic dose.

Adjuvant medications for neuropathic pain include antidepressants, anticonvulsants, corticosteroids, local anesthetics, antiarrhythmics, and certain miscellaneous medications such as baclofen, clonidine, and capsaicin cream (Table 6-2). These medications can have significant adverse effects and need to be monitored closely. Just as the opioids, they often need to be prescribed in higher than normal doses to optimize their effect. This, however, increases the risk of side effects. Because of this risk and the fact that there are limited data on the effectiveness of adjuvant drugs for analgesic purposes, health care providers are often reluctant to order adjuvant medications. This reluctance further risks poor control of cancer pain.

Antidepressants are generally the first line of adjuvant therapy for neuropathic pain. Unless contraindicated, amitriptyline (Elavil, AstraZeneca, Wilmington, Del) is the drug of choice because most studies on neuropathic pain were conducted using this drug. Contraindications for amitriptyline include cardiac arrhythmias, conduction abnormalities, narrow-angle glaucoma, and clinically significant prostatic hyperplasia. Amitriptyline is generally started at 10 to 25 mg at bedtime because sedation is a frequent side effect. Elavil can be increased by 10 mg to 25 mg every other day as needed. Because of the risk of side effects, the lowest effective dose should be used, with a maximum daily dose of 150 mg. Analgesic effect is expected in 4 to 7 days.

Anticonvulsants are most useful for lancinating, paroxysmal pain and pain that does not fully respond to antidepressant therapy. They may be used alone or in combination with antidepressants and other classifications of adjuvant analgesics. Anticonvulsants used for neuropathic pain include carbamazepine (Tegretol, Basil Pharmaceuticals, Basil, Switzerland), phenytoin (Dilantin), valproic acid (Depakote, Abbott Park, Ill), clonazepam (Klonopin, Roche, Basil, Switzerland), and gabapentin (Neurontin, Parke-Davis). Clients taking any of these anticonvulsants need to be monitored closely for side effects. Routine measurement of blood levels of these drugs is also required to monitor for toxicity. Corticosteroids have significant side effects. However, they too can relieve neuropathic pain by reducing edema that occurs with compression of nervous system structures. Steroids such as dexamethasone (Decadron, Merck, Whitehouse Station, NJ) or prednisone are recommended with opioids for the management of pain caused by brachial or lumbosacral plexopathy. Steroids are typically given in high doses during acute episodes of severe pain, then quickly tapered to avoid long-term side effects. Baclofen (Lioresal, Geigy Pharmaceuticals, Basil, Switzerland), a muscle relaxant commonly used for spasticity, potentiates relief of nerve pain and can be used in conjunction with opioids, antidepressants, antiarrhythmics, or corticosteroids. Baclofen has been found to be effective for trigeminal neuralgia as well as for other types of neuropathic pain.

Clients who are unable to tolerate adequate amounts of analgesia should be referred to a specialist who is skilled in more invasive approaches to the management of pain. Injection of local anesthetics or placement of catheters for intraspinal administration of opioids would allow higher amounts of analgesic to be delivered to the source of the pain, eliminating or decreasing the systemic effects that occur with oral or IV delivery.

SUMMARY

Individuals with cancer are at risk for a variety of physiological problems capable of causing pain. Comprehensive assessments for the etiology of the pain, appropriate treatment, and ongoing monitoring of pain are essential to achieve relief of pain and improve quality of life. Knowledge of the patterns of metastasis for cancer and the characteristics of pain are tools the physician and nurse use to identify the etiology of pain and subsequent treatment. Changes in the nature and intensity of chronic cancer pain are critical assessment findings

> Although neuropathic pain is less responsive to opioids than nociceptive pain, opioids are the first line of treatment, with morphine sulfate the drug of choice.

that require prompt medical treatment. Neuropathic pain often requires high doses of opioids along with adjunct medications to achieve relief and control of the pain. Although oral opioids and adjunct analgesics may effectively relieve neuropathic pain in some individuals, escalation of pain intensity may require rapid titration of IV opioids in a clinical setting that allows for close monitoring of side effects. Morphine continues to be the drug of choice for severe cancer pain, but high doses of morphine along with high doses of adjuvant analgesics are often required for pain relief and control.

> When pain is out of control, the route for analgesia is often changed from oral to intravenous to allow for administration of medications with a rapid onset of action.

Case Study Resolved

After receiving the order for J.T.'s admission to the hospital, the home care nurse coordinates her transfer. The nurse phones J.T. to ask when she last took MSIR. J.T. states she has not taken any morphine for 2 hours, and she denies having taken more than one tablet every 2 hours through the night. Recognizing that J.T. is not oversedated, that she does not likely have respiratory depression, that she has severe pain, and that it would take at least 30 minutes before she would be given analgesia in the hospital, the nurse instructs J.T. to take a 10 mg tablet of MSIR and to take her MSIR with her to the hospital. The nurse then calls the emergency department to give a report on J.T. and to emphasize the need for control of her intractable pain.

On arrival to the emergency department, an intravenous saline lock is inserted to administer analgesia with rapid onset of action. Analgesics given IV push will have a short half-life and will be quickly metabolized to decrease the risk of toxicity. Analgesics for J.T. are ordered according to the cancer pain emergency protocol that guides the physicians and nurses in aggressive yet safe treatment for severe pain. The protocol calls for the assessment of pain intensity (using a 0 to 10 rating scale), vital signs, level of consciousness, nausea, itching, and myoclonus (ie, twitching), which are signs of morphine toxicity.

> A cancer pain emergency protocol guides the physicians and nurses in aggressive yet safe treatment for severe pain.

A pain intensity score of 8 or higher in the absence of morphine toxicity calls for administration of morphine sulfate 10 mg IV over 15 minutes. Pain, vital signs, and signs of morphine toxicity are reassessed, and a morphine bolus is repeated 30 minutes later, the amount of which is based on the rating of pain.

The protocol used for J.T. reads that the morphine bolus is to be doubled with each successive administration (every 30 minutes) until pain is controlled, as defined by a pain severity of 5 or less on a scale of 0 to 10. Pain rated 2 to 5 in the absence of signs of toxicity is treated with a bolus dose equal to the previous dose every 30 minutes. Once the pain decreases significantly (as indicated by rating of 2 or less or statement of marked improvement), bolus doses are stopped, and a continuous morphine IV drip is instituted. The hourly rate of the drip is determined by dividing the total amount of morphine given as a bolus by two times the half-life of the drug. After receiving a total of 30 mg of morphine,

J.T. rates her pain as 0. She is started on continuous IV morphine drip at 4 mg per hour. This rate was calculated by multiplying the half-life of morphine (= 4 hours) by 2 (= 8), and dividing 8 into the total amount of drug given by bolus (ie, 30 mg/8 = 3.8 or 4 mg). Rescue PRN doses, which are 50% of the hourly rate (ie, 2 mg), are available every 20 minutes, and J.T. is monitored closely for adequacy of pain relief and development of adverse side effects.

REFERENCE

1. Cherny N, Portenoy R. The management of cancer pain. *CA: A Cancer Journal for Clinicians.* 1994;44:262-303.

BIBLIOGRAPHY

Coluzzi P. Cancer pain management: newer perspectives on opioids and episodic pain. *American Journal of Hospice and Palliative Care.* 1998;15:13-22.

Coyle N. *Neuropathic Pain.* Paper presented at Oncology Nursing Society 22nd Annual Congress, New Orleans, La; 1997.

Coyle N, Layman-Goldstein M. Pain assessment and management in palliative care. In: Matzo ML, Sherman DW, eds. *Palliative Care Nursing: Quality Care to the End of Life.* New York: Springer; 2001.

Groenwald S, Frogge M, Goodman M, Yarbro C. *Cancer Nursing Principles and Practice.* 4th ed. Boston, Mass: Jones & Bartlett; 1998.

Hagen NA, Elwood T, Ernst S. Cancer pain emergencies: a protocol for management. *J Pain Symptom Manage.* 1997;14:45-50.

Management of Cancer Pain Guidelines Panel. *Managing Cancer Pain Clinical Practice Guideline. AHCPR Pub No. 94-0595.* Rockville, Md: Agency for Health Care Policy and Research, Public Health Service, US Department of Health and Human Services; 1994.

Paice JA. Pain. In: Yarbro CH, Frogge MH, Goodman M, eds. *Cancer Symptom Management.* 2nd ed. Boston, Mass: Jones & Bartlett; 1998:118-147.

CASE STUDY QUESTIONS

1. What type of analgesic will be given to treat J.T.'s out-of-control pain?
2. Why?
3. What parameters must be monitored during administration of this medication?

MULTIPLE-CHOICE QUESTIONS

1. Nociceptive pain includes:
   A. Somatic and visceral pain
   B. Somatic and neuropathic pain
   C. Visceral and neuropathic pain
   D. Neuralgia and neuropathic pain

2. Somatic pain is characterized as well-localized, deep, dull, or achy, and originating in:
   A. Gastrointestinal structures
   B. Joint, muscle, or bone
   C. The spinal cord
   D. Peripheral nervous tissue

3. Of the following, which would most likely cause neuropathic pain?
   A. Bone metastasis
   B. Bowel obstruction
   C. Brachial plexopathy
   D. Brain tumor

4. Breakthrough pain in clients with chronic cancer should be treated with:
   A. Long-acting analgesics
   B. Short-acting analgesics
   C. Analgesics with a long half-life
   D. Adjuvant medications

5. Which of the following side effects occurs most often when opioids are increased for chronic cancer pain?
   A. Respiratory depression
   B. Sedation
   C. Vomiting
   D. Opioid toxicity

6. Which of the following adjunct medications is an antidepressant that is commonly used for neuropathic pain?
   A. Acetaminophen
   B. Amitriptyline
   C. Dexamethasone
   D. Phenytoin

CASE STUDY ANSWERS

1. The analgesic should be a narcotic that is a.) potent; b.) fast acting; c.) with a short half-life; d.) without a ceiling. Depending on the setting and other specifics, the route will be oral or intravenous.

2. Although adjuvant medications are often helpful in treatment of neuropathic pain, a narcotic analgesic is the first step. The narcotic analgesic should be potent because the pain is severe. Neuropathic pain often requires high doses of narcotic analgesics. The analgesic should be fast acting because the goal is to relieve the pain as soon as possible. The analgesic should have a short half-life to avoid accumulation and drug toxicity. The analgesic should not have a ceiling because J.T.'s pain has already been shown to require more than 60 mg of morphine each 24 hours and will likely require more. Choosing a drug without a ceiling eliminates the need to limit analgesia because of dose. Morphine is usually used initially because health care practitioners have had the most experience with it.

3. Parameters to monitor include level of pain, vital signs, sedation, nausea, itching, and myoclonus.

MULTIPLE-CHOICE ANSWERS

1. A
2. B
3. C
4. B
5. B
6. B

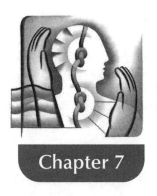

Chapter 7

Pain in the Adult With HIV

Case Study

T.D. is a 32-year-old female who has had human immunodeficiency virus (HIV) for 5 years. She believes that she was exposed to HIV through shared needles when she abused intravenous drugs. She presents to the clinic with recent onset of mouth pain but has no fever or dental problems. When asked about the presence of other symptoms of discomfort, she admits that she continues to have her usual headaches, which have not changed in frequency or intensity. She states that the muscle aches in her legs occur less frequently and are less intense than previously. She denies having the burning or tingling that she experienced in her feet when taking didanosine (ddI; Videx, Bristol Myers Squibb, New York, NY) last year. Since stopping the ddI, she states she has been following her new medication regimen faithfully. At the present time, she is taking a combination protocol of antiretroviral agents that includes two nucleoside reverse transcriptase inhibitors (zidovudine and lamivudine) and one protease inhibitor (saquinavir).

PREVALENCE OF PAIN RELATED TO HIV INFECTION

Statistics on the prevalence of pain in clients with HIV infection vary, but it is known that pain can occur at any point throughout the HIV trajectory. A study reported in 1993[1] found that 53 (28%) of 191 seropositive men with asymptomatic disease had HIV-related pain. In 1998, Breibart[2] reported that 40% to 60% of clients with HIV had pain.

Studies on clients with acquired immunodeficiency syndrome (AIDS) indicate that pain is present in 50% to 80% of clients, and that pain in this group is more severe than at earlier stages.[3] Pain related to HIV infection is often compared to pain related to cancer in terms of its prevalence, intensity, impact on quality of life, treatment, and undertreatment.

In terms of intensity, HIV-related pain is considered comparable to pain experienced in clients with cancer. Intensity of the pain also increases with progression of HIV, as it does with cancer. The client with HIV commonly has two to three pains at a time, whereas the client with cancer has an average of three. As seen in clients with cancer, pain in clients with HIV also has an enormously negative impact on an individual's quality of life. It can lead to functional disabilities, social isolation, depression, hopelessness, and suicidal ideation. Comprehensive assessment of the physiological, psychological, sociocultural, developmental, and spiritual dimensions of a client's life is necessary to adequately address pain related to either cancer or HIV.

ETIOLOGIES OF PAIN RELATED TO HIV INFECTION

Pain associated with HIV can be related to:
1. The virus itself
2. An opportunistic infection or malignancy secondary to HIV
3. Treatment of the virus or related illnesses
4. Pathology unrelated to HIV

In terms of duration, HIV-related pain may be acute or chronic. Acute or short-term pain is directly related to tissue injury and resolves with tissue healing. An example of short-term pain related to an opportunistic infection is pain in the oropharynx due to candidiasis (ie, fungus). An example of short-term pain related to treatment for HIV is abdominal pain from acute pancreatitis, which is a side effect of certain antiretroviral agents such as ddI (didanosine) and ddC (zalcitabine).

Chronic pain can occur secondary to tissue healing, HIV pathology (ie, damage to tissue caused by the virus itself), chronic infections, malignancies secondary to HIV, or as a side effect of medications such as antiretrovirals. Chronic pain may be persistent or episodic. A classification system for chronic HIV-related pain based on the pain type and its etiology is currently being developed, but it is not complete owing to the relative newness of the HIV epidemic and evolving knowledge on this topic.

Chronic HIV-related pain is classified as visceral, somatic, or neuropathic depending on its physiological etiology and the quality of the pain. Somatic pain arises from bones, muscles, joints, or skin, and is often described as aching, throbbing, or stabbing. Skin pain is often described as burning. Visceral pain that arises from gastrointestinal structures often varies with the structures involved and is referred to common cutaneous sites. Obstruction of a hollow viscous is associated with cramping or gnawing pain. Injury to other visceral organs is characterized by aching, stabbing, or throbbing pain. Neuropathic pain originates from the central or peripheral nervous system and is characterized as sharp, burning, shooting, shock-like, or electric. Although neuropathic pain is common in HIV-infected clients, it does not represent the majority of pain in this client population. Pains of somatic and visceral etiology comprise the majority of HIV-related pain. All three types of pain can also occur at the same time.

COMMON SYNDROMES OF PAIN WITH HIV INFECTION

As of 1996, the most common syndromes of pain related to HIV include headache, arthralgias, myalgias, painful peripheral neuropathy, pharyngeal pain, abdominal pain, painful dermatological conditions, and pain due to extensive Kaposi's sarcoma.

The most common syndromes of pain related to HIV include headaches, arthralgias, myalgias, painful peripheral neuropathy, pharyngeal pain, abdominal pain, painful dermatological conditions, and pain due to extensive Kaposi's sarcoma.

Headaches

Headaches are prevalent in HIV-infected clients, and they occur more frequently in women. HIV-related headaches could be caused by infections (eg, bacterial sinusitis, cryptococcal or toxoplasmosis meningitis), malignancy (eg, lymphoma), or medications (eg, zidovudine, didanosine, indinavir). Headaches may also be an exacerbation of a pre-existing migraine or tension headache syndrome. New onset or increased intensity of a headache should be evaluated promptly by a physician to rule out a life-threatening cause. The incidence of headaches secondary to antiretroviral therapy increases with certain combination therapy regimens for HIV. One clinical trial[4] of 196 clients compared taking zidovudine, zidovudine combined with indinavir, and indinavir alone. The incidence of headaches increased from 5.6% to 11.7% when both zidovudine and indinavir were taken. The same study showed that the incidence of headaches decreased to 5.1% when indinavir was taken alone. A clinical trial[5] of 230 clients taking zidovudine and lamivudine found that the incidence of headaches increased from 27% in clients taking zidovudine alone to 35% in those taking these drugs together.

Individuals with headaches secondary to antiretroviral therapy should have their medication regimen monitored by physicians and nurses experienced with these drugs to evaluate the benefits of the therapy given the adverse effects.

Treatment of headaches involves treating the underlying cause and providing symptomatic support. Individuals with headaches secondary to antiretroviral therapy should have their medication regimen monitored by physicians and nurses who are experienced with these drugs to evaluate the benefits of the therapy given the adverse effects. The effects of combination antiretroviral therapy on decreasing HIV-RNA levels and increasing CD4 levels in clients with HIV have been significant. To maximize their chances for increased survival, clients may elect to continue experiencing certain side effects such as headaches.

Clients experiencing headaches secondary to antiretroviral therapy should be provided with analgesics, the potency of which is based on the severity and the frequency of the pain. Acetaminophen on an as-needed basis may be sufficient for headaches of mild intensity. A more potent medication such as oxycodone or oxycodone acetaminophen combination (eg, Percocet, Tylox) should be offered for headaches of moderate to severe intensity. Clients who do not obtain adequate relief from this or any other medication should be evaluated for a possible change to another narcotic. Changes in antiretroviral regimens also depend on each client's tolerance to side effects and ability to adhere to treatment plans.

Clients with HIV-related headaches might also benefit from nonpharmacological interventions used in conjunction with medications. Resting in a dark and quiet environment with a cold washcloth or ice bag placed on the forehead could facilitate relief. Frontal headaches secondary to sinus congestion may improve with warmth and steam. Headaches originating at the back of the head or neck often represent muscle tension as a source. Heat and massage, acupressure, and reflexology (massage limited to the feet or hands only) can be effective for muscle tension.

Pharyngeal Pain

Pharyngeal pain that causes difficulty swallowing is usually related to fungal infections, herpes simplex, or Kaposi's sarcoma. Other causes include ulcerative lesions of infectious or nonspecific origins. Treatment of pharyngeal pain involves treating the underlying cause and providing symptomatic support. Local or systemic antifungal agents are prescribed for infections suspected to be fungal. Acyclovir is prescribed if the lesions appear like vesicles (ie, herpetic).

Muscle and Joint Pain

Several arthritis and arthralgia syndromes related to HIV infection and HIV- related illnesses are known to cause chronic somatic pain in joints, muscles, and other tissues. Examples of these syndromes include an HIV-associated arthritis, nonspecific arthralgias, Reiter's syndrome, and psoriatic arthritis. A septic myositis and HIV-associated myositis can also occur. Arthralgias and myalgias that cause chronic somatic pain also occur as a side effect of antiviral drugs such as zidovudine. Myopathy characterized by muscle weakness, elevated creatinine kinase, myalgia, and cramping can occur secondary to HIV infection, microsporidia, zidovudine, isoniazid (INH), alcohol, or illicit drugs.

Peripheral Neuropathy

Up to 50% of clients infected with HIV experience some degree of painful neuropathy, with the severity and course of the pain varying greatly. A generalized neuropathy may be caused by the virus itself; by HIV-related illnesses such as cytomegalovirus, herpes zoster, or mycobacterium; or by medications, alcohol, or vitamin deficiencies (eg, B_6, B_{12}). Medications used in treatment of HIV that cause peripheral neuropathy include certain antiretroviral agents (eg, ddI, ddC, stavudine), certain anti-infective agents (eg, metronidazole, isoniazid, rifampin, ethionamide), medications to treat cytomegalovirus (eg, foscarnet), medications to prevent *Pneumocystis carinii* pneumonia (eg, dapsone), and medications to treat Kaposi's sarcoma (eg, vincristine, vinblastine). If the cause of the peripheral neuropathy is thought to be a medication, the dose of the medication is decreased or the drug may be stopped. Tricyclic antidepressants are the drugs of choice to treat peripheral neuropathy, but individuals with HIV infection can be very sensitive to these drugs. Drug levels of these medications should be monitored closely. Opioids may also be used to treat pain related to peripheral neuropathy. In 1998, Breitbart,[2] an expert in the management of HIV-related pain, stated that the increased use of protease inhibitors is preventing the development of severe pain related to HIV and AIDS, but that significant improvement in peripheral neuropathy is not being observed using these drugs.

Abdominal Pain

Abdominal pain in a client with HIV infection can be caused by enteritis, cholecystitis, hepatitis, pancreatitis, organomegaly, or tumor invasion of organs. Recurrent abdominal pain with diarrhea can be a result of opportunistic bacterial, viral, or parasitic infections; HIV infection; antiviral therapy; or antibiotic therapy.

Dermatological Pain

Clients with Kaposi's sarcoma can experience severe pain due to direct infiltration of the tumors into the skin or to associated lymphedema. Treatment of pain would include chemotherapy to treat the Kaposi's sarcoma and narcotic analgesics.

ANALGESICS FOR HIV-RELATED PAIN

Treatment of pain related to HIV infection ideally should be aimed at treating the cause of the pain. However, treatment of the cause does not always alleviate the pain, and identification of the cause is not always possible. Adequate treatment of HIV-related pain frequently requires the use of pharmacological agents on either a short- or long-term basis. Treatment for HIV-related pain should be fundamentally the same as the treatment of cancer pain and should be guided by the Agency for Health Care Policy and Research (AHCPR) *Clinical Practice Guidelines for Management of Cancer Pain.*[6] These guidelines promote use of the World Health Organization (WHO) analgesic ladder, which bases treatment on the severity of the pain. Nonopioid analgesics should be used for mild pain and opioid analgesics for moderate to severe pain. Morphine sulfate is considered the drug of choice for moderate to severe pain, with the oral route and controlled-release medications being the most widely used. Adjuvant medications should be used in addition to an opioid for neuropathic pain. Other principles of pain management that guide treatment of HIV-related pain (as well as cancer) described in the AHCPR guidelines include recommendations to give around-the-clock medications to prevent chronic pain and short-acting analgesics for breakthrough pain. The AHCPR guidelines also recommend the use of equianalgesic conversions, use of a variety of interventions to control pain (eg, complementary therapies such as massage, imagery, therapeutic touch) and comprehensive assessments and treatments that address the multidimensional aspects of the person (eg, physiological, psychosocial, spiritual, developmental).

COMPLEMENTARY THERAPIES FOR HIV-RELATED PAIN

Regardless of the cause, clients with chronic pain often benefit from the practice of complementary therapies used in conjunction with pharmacological interventions. Clients with HIV are no exception to this rule. In fact, surveys indicate that up to 70% of clients infected with HIV have sought some form of alternative or complementary therapy.[7] Complementary or alternative therapies are particularly appropriate for use in this client population because of their enhancing effect on the immune system and their low risk for adverse effects. Examples of complementary therapies shown to alleviate pain in clients with HIV include chiropractic, osteopathic, and massage therapies for musculoskeletal symptoms and peripheral neuropathies, and therapeutic touch for peripheral neuropathies and other HIV-associated pain.

CHAPTER SUMMARY

Assessing for the etiology of pain in clients with HIV is particularly challenging because opportunistic diseases, malignancies, and treatments cause pain in so many systems of the body; and the cause of each pain is not always identifiable. The goals in assessing pain related to HIV infection are to identify new symptoms of pain promptly and to rule in or rule out the cause of the pain so that treatment can be promptly initiated. This is particularly important when infection is the cause of one's pain. Infections are life-threatening to clients with HIV, and initiation of appropriate treatment may be essential to keeping the client alive or maintaining quality of life.

Physicians specializing in infectious disease who are knowledgeable about the complexities of HIV disease and HIV treatment should be consulted for painful syndromes of unknown causes. It is sometimes said "to know HIV is to know all of medicine," and arriving at a diagnosis in a person with this illness often requires the expertise of someone who frequently deals with the disease and its ever-evolving treatment.

Infection with HIV puts an individual at high risk for experiencing a variety of pain syndromes. Knowledge of the common symptoms and patterns of pain related to HIV infection assists health care providers in identifying the cause, significance, and treatment for the pain. Because pain can indicate a life-threatening infection, malignancy, or reaction to a drug, each new pain should be recognized as potentially significant and, if necessary, the client should be referred to an infection control specialist with expertise in HIV.

Antiretroviral therapy, the mainstay of treatment for HIV infection, commonly causes painful syndromes such as headaches and peripheral neuropathy. Because adherence to antiretroviral schedules is vital to optimal treatment for HIV infection, clients need to be monitored closely for their tolerance and willingness to take these medications. Clients with HIV-related pain should also be provided with pharmacological and nonpharmacological strategies to assist in pain control.

> Adherence to antiretroviral schedules is vital to optimal treatment for HIV infection. Patients need to be monitored closely for their tolerance and willingness to take these medications.

Pain in the client with HIV can be related to a variety of causes, and information on treatment of pain continues to evolve. Consequently, medication management of HIV is complex, and recommendations for treatment of the disease and related complications can quickly change. It is essential that physicians and nurses caring for clients with HIV monitor for signs and symptoms of pain related to HIV, and frequently confer with experts in the field to maximize client outcomes.

Case Study Resolved

The fact that T.D. is infected with HIV and knowledge of patterns of pain with HIV infection alerts the health care provider to her report of mouth pain, headaches, and leg pain. Additional information about the location, character, intensity, and treatment of her headaches and leg pain is obtained, and a targeted physical assessment of her oral cavity and neurological system is performed. Findings of this assessment are evaluated in view of her current medications and past history.

Assessment of the oral cavity reveals creamy, white plaques on the tongue and buccal mucosa. Based on her history of oral candida, the health care provider believes that recurrent oral candidiasis is responsible for T.D.'s mouth pain. Treatment of the cause of the pain (the candidiasis) with Nystatin suspension, lozenges, or other antifungal agents such as clotrimazole or fluconazole should relieve the oral pain as the candida clears. The goal of treatment for candidiasis is complete resolution of the lesions and pain. It is important that T.D. be able to tolerate a full course of treatment to achieve complete resolution. Dislike for the taste of an antifungal suspension could risk nonadherence and incomplete response. The health care provider assesses the client's willingness to follow through with liquid antifungal treatment and offers an antifungal agent in pill form if necessary. (Ketoconazole increases saquinavir drug levels three-fold and is not the drug of choice.)

T.D.'s report of headache is significant because of her risk for infectious meningitis and lymphoma, both of which can manifest as headaches. If her headache was new in onset, was associated with fever, or had increased in frequency and intensity, it would likely be more of a concern. Her record states that she has been having occasional frontal headaches over the last 3 months, which her physician attributes to the antiretroviral therapy (zidovudine and lamivudine). T.D. states that she occasionally takes two tablets of acetaminophen to relieve her headaches and that she tolerates the occasional headaches well. She also states that she is willing to continue her current antiviral therapy despite her headaches and that she will notify the physician if they increase in frequency or intensity, or if she needs a stronger analgesic.

The fact that T.D. no longer has burning and tingling in her feet suggests that this pain (which she had last year) represented peripheral neuropathy, likely caused by didanosine. When T.D. experienced this in the past, she admitted that she stopped taking her didanosine (ddI) because she could not tolerate the pain. T.D.'s inability to follow a medication regimen with ddI prompts the change in antiretroviral therapy to a regimen with less risk for neuropathy and nonadherence to the medication schedule. Once T.D. stopped taking ddI, the peripheral neuropathy resolves and she faithfully follows the new antiviral regimen.

The fact that T.D.'s muscle pain in her legs has decreased in frequency likely represents better control of the HIV itself, which is often the cause of such muscle discomfort. Since she changed from her past antiretroviral therapy to the current therapy with the protease inhibitor saquinavir, her viral load has decreased significantly.

Discussion of T.D.'s pain would not be complete without mention of the potential effect pain has on the psychosocial and other dimensions of life, and the effect that these dimensions have on her pain. It is important to recognize that pain in women with HIV infection is twice as likely to be undertreated than pain in men, and that pain in clients with HIV infection and a history of drug abuse is 1.8 times as likely to be undertreated.[3] Although nurses do not prescribe analgesics, they play a major role in the treatment of pain. Nurses advocating for clients with pain should understand that injustices in the treatment of pain based on gender and histories of drug abuse exist and interfere with effective treatment and quality of life. Studies looking at the use of analgesia for HIV-related pain indicate that clients with histories of drug abuse do not use more analgesics than those without histories of drug abuse.[3] Nurses and health care providers should not be distracted with concerns about possible abuse of analgesics in this client population. They should, instead, focus their efforts on relieving the client's pain, regardless of personal history.

If the correct analgesia for HIV-related pain is chosen, clients will achieve relief of pain 75% to 80% of the time.[3] In some clients, the source of pain is not identifiable, despite a comprehensive work-up. The inability to identify the source of pain in a client with HIV is

> Patients with HIV-related pain should achieve relief of pain 75% to 80% of the time.

not uncommon, and it is not an appropriate reason for withholding pain medication. The potential and actual effects of inadequate treatment of pain on the client's quality of life should guide the treatment of pain, regardless of the cause or the circumstances.

REFERENCES

1. Singer E, Surlier C, Fahy-Chandon B, Chi S, Syndulko K, Tourtellotte W. Painful symptoms reported by HIV-infected men in a longitudinal study. *Pain.* 1993;54:15-19.
2. Breitbart W. *Pain Management in HIV/AIDS.* Paper presented at the 9th National Meeting for State Cancer Pain Initiatives, Portland, Me; 1998.

3. Breitbart W. Pharmacotherapy of pain in AIDS. In: Wormser GP, ed. *A Clinical Guide to AIDS and HIV*. Philadelphia, Pa: Lippincott-Raven; 1996:359-378.

4. Merck Laboratories. Crixivan (indinavir sulfate). West Point, Pa: Merck; 1996.

5. GlaxoWellcome. Epivir (lamivudine) in combination with Retrovir (zidovudine). Research Triangle Park, NC: GlaxoWellcome; 1995.

6. Management of Cancer Pain Guideline Panel. *Management of Cancer Pain Clinical Practice Guideline. AHCPR Pub No. 94-0592*. Rockville, Md: Agency for Health Care Policy and Research, Public Health Service, US Department of Health and Human Services; 1994.

7. Evans BM. Complementary therapies and HIV infection. *Am J Nurs*. 1999;99(2):42-45.

BIBLIOGRAPHY

Breitbart W, Rosenfeld BD, Passik SD, McDonald MV, Thaler H, Portenoy R. The undertreatment of pain in ambulatory AIDS patients. *Pain*. 1996;65(2/3):243-249.

Newshan MA. Therapeutic touch for symptom control in persons with AIDS. *Holistic Nursing Practice*. 1989;3(4):45-51.

Portenoy RK. *Pain in Oncologic and AIDS Patients*. Newtown, Pa: Handbooks in Health Care; 1997.

CASE STUDY QUESTIONS

1. What is the likely cause of T.D.'s muscle aches?
2. What is the likely cause of T.D.'s headache?
3. What did the burning and tingling in T.D.'s feet likely represent?
4. What was the likely cause of the pain syndrome manifested by burning and tingling?
5. What are possible causes of T.D.'s mouth pain?

MULTIPLE-CHOICE QUESTIONS

1. In clients with HIV, headaches of moderate intensity that are not relieved by acetaminophen should be treated with:
    A. Aspirin
    B. Ibuprofen
    C. Morphine
    D. Oxycodone

2. Recommended nonpharmacological interventions for headaches related to HIV:
    A. Are not as effective as medications
    B. Are more effective than medications
    C. Should be used in conjunction with medications
    D. Should not be used in conjunction with antiretrovirals

3. Antiretrovirals that are most often responsible for pain-related peripheral neuropathy include:
    A. Didanosine (ddI), zalcitabine (ddC), and stavudine
    B. Indinovir and ddI
    C. Lamiduvine and indinovir
    D. Zidovudine (AZT) and lamiduvine

4. The class of medications that is considered the preferred treatment for painful peripheral neuropathy in clients with HIV is:
    A. Antiretrovirals
    B. Protease inhibitors
    C. Tricyclic antidepressants
    D. Nonsteroidal anti-inflammatory drugs (NSAIDs)

5. A "new" symptom of pain in a client with HIV should be:
    A. Fully assessed and reported to the physician
    B. Monitored while withholding treatment
    C. Treated with analgesics
    D. Treated with complementary therapies

CASE STUDY ANSWERS

1. Somatic pain such as muscle aches often occur in HIV-infected individuals. They may be associated with nonspecific arthralgias or myalgias, or may occur as a side effect of zidovudine. The fact that T.D.'s muscle pain has decreased supports the fact that the virus itself was responsible for the muscle pain.

2. Headaches in a patient with HIV infection may be related to a central nervous system infection or malignancy. Once these causes are ruled out, antiretroviral therapy is often considered to be the cause. Headaches are often a side effect of taking zidovudine, didanosine, indinavir, and/or lamivudine. T.D. is currently taking zidovudine and lamivudine. The incidence of headaches in patients taking zidovudine and lamivudine is significantly higher than for patients taking zidovudine alone.

3. Peripheral neuropathy.

4. The antiretroviral drug didanosine (ddI, Videx) can cause peripheral neuropathy. T.D. was taking didanosine when she had the burning and tingling in her feet. The burning and tingling resolved after she stopped taking ddI.

5. Causes of mouth pain in a person with HIV infection include fungal infections, herpes simplex, and Kaposi's sarcoma.

MULTIPLE-CHOICE ANSWERS

1. D. Acetaminophen on an as-needed basis may be sufficient for headaches of mild intensity. A more potent medication such as oxycodone or an oxycodone and acetaminophen combination should be offered for headaches of moderate to severe intensity.

2. C. Heat, cold, massage, acupressure, and reflexology have been recommended to be used in conjunction with medication.

3. A. Certain antiretrovirals used in the treatment of HIV cause peripheral neuropathy. These include ddI, ddC, and stavudine.

4. C. Opioids may be used to treat pain related to peripheral neuropathy but tricyclic antidepressants are the drugs of choice.

5. A. New symptoms of pain in clients with HIV must be promptly assessed to rule in or rule out the cause. This is particularly important because an infectious etiology can be life-threatening. Initiation of appropriate treatment may be essential to keeping the client alive or maintaining quality of life.

Chapter 8

Chronic Back Pain in Adults

Case Study

Mrs. K. is a 30-year-old woman who works as a registered nurse in a community hospital. While assisting a client during a cardiac arrest, she injures her lower back. Mrs. K. is examined by an orthopedic surgeon, who finds no neurological deficits and no significant abnormalities on radiographic study of the spine. A diagnosis of lumbosacral strain is made, and Mrs. K. is provided with a plan of care consisting of bedrest for 3 days, ibuprofen 400 mg every 6 hours, cyclobenzaprine (Flexeril, Merck) 10 mg three times a day, and moist heat as needed. She is also instructed not to return to work or perform strenuous activity (eg, lifting) until she is seen and cleared by the physician.

For more than 1 week, Mrs. K. remains on bedrest, walking to the bathroom as needed. Her pain initially improves with rest, so she continues to limit her activity as much as possible. She states she is afraid that any increase in her activity will cause disc herniation. She stops taking her cyclobenzaprine but increases the dose of nonsteroidal anti-inflammatory medication to 600 mg every 6 hours.

On follow-up visits with her physician 4 and 8 weeks after injury, she informs the physician that her pain continues and that she has pain in her buttocks. He tells her that there is no evidence of a disc disorder and that she can return to work for 4-hour periods. There is no discussion about her pain experience, and no other recommendations for treatment or symptom relief are made.

When Mrs. K. returns to work, she finds that she is extremely stiff, with dull pain in her low back after 4 hours. After several days of work, much of her stiffness is relieved, but her pain continues. Ten weeks after injury, the orthopedic surgeon tells her she may return to work full-time and releases her from his care. Out of frustration, Mrs. K. makes an appointment with her internist, who tells her there is nothing wrong neurologically and gives her a handout with instructions for pelvic tilt exercises. Mrs. K. performs the exercises as prescribed by the physician but finds that it does not help relieve the pain. Frustrated and concerned that she may not be performing the exercises properly, she refers herself to a physical therapist who is described as someone with expertise in back pain. The therapist urges Mrs. K. to increase the number of pelvic tilts she is doing and gives her a few additional exercises to strengthen her back. ⁻

Mrs. K. finds that one of the exercises (upper trunk extension) helps relieve her pain, but that the pelvic tilt (a flexion exercise) actually causes an intensity in the pain. Because she is concerned she will harm herself further, Mrs. K. stops doing the pelvic tilts. On sharing this information with the therapist, the therapist tells Mrs. K. that there is nothing more she can do for her if she is not going to do her exercises.

Concerned that she is not improving, Mrs. K. again contacts her internist to request a computed tomography (CT scan). Before this is ordered, she is required to see her physician, who reassesses her neurological status and finds no deficits. The physician agrees to order a CT scan, which is performed 1 week later. Three weeks after the scan, the physician notifies Mrs. K. that the CT findings are normal. He gives her no further recommendations to help her with her pain.

CAUSES OF LOW BACK PAIN

The causes of low back pain are many and varied. In most clients, degenerative disc disease (officially termed *spondylosis*) is an underlying factor. Muscular and ligament inflammation is the cause of low back pain in another large percentage of Americans. In the remaining clients, low back pain is generally related to complications of other diseases such as cancer, infection, rheumatic disorders, or other conditions, many of which are rare.

Specific causes of low back pain are difficult to diagnose. Radiographic studies (x-rays) will show the bony anatomy of the spine, but soft tissues are not well-visualized. Therefore, fractures, tumors, and congenital abnormalities may be ruled in or ruled out, but these are not the major causes of low back pain. Degenerative disc disease is often seen on x-rays, but simply finding evidence of this on x-ray does not explain back pain because degenerative disease occurs in almost half the population and most of these people are asymptomatic. Diagnostic tests such as magnetic resonance imaging (MRI) are more valuable for diagnosing soft tissue, muscle, and ligament abnormalities. However, MRIs are not routinely performed on clients with acute low back pain but are generally reserved for clients who have back pain lasting more than 1 month that does not respond to treatment.

When diagnostic tests, physical examination findings, and the client's history rule in or rule out certain abnormalities, more specific diagnoses for low back pain can be made. Diagnostic labels (Table 8-1) for specific types of degenerative disc disease or muscular or ligamentous causes of low back pain include:
1. Lumbosacral strain or sprain
2. Disc herniation
3. Discogenic syndrome
4. Spondylolisthesis
5. Facet syndrome
6. Spinal stenosis
7. Spinal instability

Table 8-1

Diagnostic Labels for Low Back Pain

Disc herniation: herniation or displacement of the nucleus pulposus partly or completely through a defect in the annulus from the intervertebral space into the spinal canal or foramen or outside the foramen.

Discogenic syndrome: imprecise term that suggests annulus tears and release of a chemical mediator from the lumbar disc, resulting in pain.

Facet syndrome: pain in the facets, also referred to as zygapophyseal joints; this pain is located only in the back and is aggravated by movement, particularly rotation, and improves with rest.

Lumbosacral strain or sprain: muscular and ligamentous injury.

Spinal stenosis: old term describing the condition when the spinal canal is narrowed either congenitally or from spondylosis.

Spinal instability: occurs when movement of bony elements is identified on flexion or extension, on motion films, or in repeated studies. The definition is controversial.

Spondylolysis: a structural defect in the pars interarticularis.

Spondylolisthesis: slipping of one vertebral segment onto another.

Spondylosis: general term that describes all the changes that occur with degenerative disc disease, including desiccation of the disc, narrowing of the interspace, inflammatory and degenerative changes in the bone, ligament hypertrophy, and bone spurring.

Adapted from Long DM. *Contemporary Diagnosis and Management of Pain.* Newton, Pa: Handbooks in Health Care; 1997.

Because evidence to support one of these specific diagnoses is often lacking, low back pain is frequently described in terms of its duration (eg, acute versus chronic) and site (eg, lumbosacral spine), as opposed to its cause.

ACUTE LOW BACK PAIN

Low back pain is one of the two most common complaints of Americans, equal in incidence only to headaches.[1] Low back pain has occurred in at least 60% of American adults, with an incidence of 30%. At any one point in time, 10% to 12% of Americans are actively seeking treatment for back pain.

Most occurrences of low back pain are acute, self-limiting, and benign, lasting less than 1 month.[2] Some occurrences last longer, but most resolve within 3 months.

> Most occurrences of low back pain are acute, self-limiting, benign, and last less than 1 month.

A history and physical examination, with an emphasis on the severity of pain and neurological function below the level of the pain, should be performed. Severe pain or pain considered to be related to trauma, metastatic disease, or neurological dysfunction will likely prompt the physician to obtain x-rays of the spine, MRI, and a consultation with a

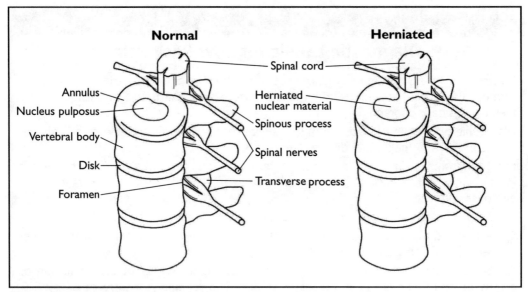

Figure 8-1. Herniated nucleus pulposus.

back specialist. A CT scan may be of some value in diagnosing the source of pain, but CT scans are limited by the fact that they do not show soft tissue injury. MRI is often the test of choice because it not only shows soft tissue injury, but also shows disc herniation with great accuracy. Bony anatomy, however, is seen better on CT scan than on plain x-rays.

Unless pain is severe without alleviation after medication or rest, or related to significant trauma or a malignancy, imagery studies (ie, CT scan or MRI) are generally not required for acute back pain. Back pain of acute origin is expected to resolve in days or weeks. Imaging studies are reasonable, however, for back pain lasting 1 month or longer, but they do not consistently identify the pathology.

Most causes of acute low back pain originate within muscles or ligaments of the back. Diagnostic labels related to acute low back pain include:
1. Lumbosacral strain or sprain
2. Disc herniation
3. Injury to zygapophyseal joints
4. Minor annular tears

A lumbosacral strain or sprain implies a muscle or ligament injury, similar to an ankle sprain. A diagnosis of disc herniation should be made only when the nucleus pulposus has been displaced (or herniates) partly or completely from the intervertebral space through a defect in the annulus into the spinal canal or foramen or outside the foramen (Figure 8-1). True disc herniation is actually a rare cause of back pain, but clients with herniated discs typically have had previous episodes of acute back pain. There is some evidence that over time a disc can work its way through an annulus before the final herniation occurs.

A degenerated disc is one that has no herniation, but the entire nucleus has undergone drying and degeneration. Although degenerative disc disease is a common cause, acute low back pain can also occur secondary to bony fracture, ligamentous disruption of a joint, or an annular tear. These causes are considered particularly when there is a history of trauma or injury.

Clients with acute low back pain often do not present themselves to a health care provider until pain significantly interferes with their activity. The examination and work-up focus on ruling in or out a cause that requires immediate treatment for an actual or potential neurological deficit. Clients with nerve root compression related to a herniated disc or trauma may undergo surgery within days of onset of pain.

If neurological deficits are not involved, immediate surgery for back pain is generally not necessary. The goal for the majority of clients with acute low back pain is to decrease inflammation and pain. Bedrest limited to 3 days or less and combinations of anti-inflammatory drugs, analgesics, and muscle relaxants are ordered to accomplish these goals. Use of opioid analgesics for a few days may be required for some episodes of acute back pain. The use of hot or cold applications to the back can also enhance back comfort for some clients. Heat, passive physical therapy, massage, and ultrasound may be performed, but these treatments have shown only temporary improvement of acute low back pain.

Most clients with acute low back pain are incapacitated no longer than 1 or 2 weeks. They benefit from returning to their level of activity as soon as it is tolerated. Identification of activities that aggravate the client's pain is important to assist the client in making modifications to reduce aggravation of the injury. With recovery from pain, an exercise program is developed in conjunction with the client to help prevent recurrence.

Because acute back pain is such a common and significant problem, the Agency for Health Care Policy and Research (AHCPR) brought together a panel of experts who collected and reviewed data on prescribed treatment plans for this problem. AHCPR guidelines for acute low back problems in adults were published in 1995 to standardize medical interventions, allowing the best chance for an optimal outcome.

Any client with back pain lasting 3 months or longer should have a full physical examination to rule in or out systemic causes of the pain (eg, malignancy). Persistent low back syndrome that is manifested by pain in the back or leg can vary in intensity, generally does not improve spontaneously, and may linger for years.

CHRONIC LOW BACK PAIN

Causes of chronic low back pain fall into one of three general categories:
1. Degenerative disc disease (spondylosis)
2. Myofascial pain
3. Other (eg, rheumatoid arthritis, metastatic cancer, or complications related to a systemic illness)

Clients with degenerative disc disease make up approximately 60% of chronic back pain cases. Degenerative disc disease changes that often lead to chronic pain involve spurring with nerve root compression, instability, facet joint disease, disc herniation, or spinal stenosis.

Causes of chronic low back pain fall into one of three general categories:
1. Degenerative disc disease
2. Myofascial pain
3. Other (eg, rheumatoid arthritis, metastatic cancer, or complications related to a systemic illness)

Twenty percent of chronic low back pain is related to myofascial pain. Myofascial pain is characteristically generalized, radiating to hips, buttocks, groin, and upper thighs. The radiation of pain, however, does not suggest or represent nerve root compression such as that which occurs with herniation. The hallmark of myofascial pain is the discovery of specific areas of inflammation in the muscles, referred to as trigger points. Trigger points can often be palpated in deep muscle as small, hard, painful knots. These triggers are thought to occur either primary or secondary to prolonged muscle spasm. Common locations of trigger points related to low back pain involve the paravertebral muscles or the glutei, and less often the thigh muscles and the area over the greater trochanter.

> The hallmark of myofascial pain is the discovery of specific areas of inflammation in the muscles, referred to as trigger points.

> Trigger points often can be palpated in deep muscle as small, hard, painful knots.

Acute low back pain that persists longer than 2 to 3 months is often described as chronic or persistent back pain. Although there is no clear-cut point where acute back pain can be labeled chronic, the transition from acute to chronic most likely occurs before a period of 6 months. Persistent low back pain is now recognized as different than pain associated with acute back pain that diminishes and resolves. Persistent low back syndrome or chronic benign pain involves similar processes as in acute pain, including nerve irritation, muscle spasm, and/or inflammation in the peripheral tissues and central nervous system (spinal cord and brain). Chronic pain, however, differs from acute pain in that it lacks the normal checks and balances that serve to dampen or modulate acute pain processes. The alterations in these checks and balances can also perpetuate the pain signal and are thought to be responsible for pain that occurs even after tissue heals and pain that often occurs outside an area of injury.

Treatment of Chronic Low Back Pain

Treatment of chronic back pain depends on identification of the cause of the pain, but a thorough understanding of all causes is lacking. Therefore, treatment of chronic back pain is often limited to situations in which a definitive cause can be identified. Even if the cause is identified, treatment is not consistently effective. Researchers continue to collect information on chronic inflammation, muscle spasms, central nervous system mechanisms, and chronic pain mechanisms in an effort to improve treatment options and effectiveness.

Chronic pain related to inflammation, muscles, or nerve involvement may be treated with anti-inflammatory medications, muscle relaxants, anticonvulsants, and antidepressants as described under acute pain management. Chronic pain related to malignancy is commonly treated with opioids and nonsteroidal anti-inflammatory medications, both given around the clock (versus as-needed).

Treatment of myofascial pain involves local heat, massage, transcutaneous electrical nerve stimulation (TENS), and injections of saline, anesthetic, or a corticosteroid directly into the muscle. Injections may need to be repeated over days to weeks. Treatment of myofascial pain generally requires a health care provider with a specialty in pain management. Once myofascial pain is controlled, clients should be guided through an exercise program to strengthen the involved muscles and avoid future pain.

Table 8-2

Barriers to Effective Treatment of Chronic Back Pain

Limited knowledge about the pathology
Medical education on chronic benign back pain is limited
Western medicine offers limited treatment options
Clients are not aware of lack of standardization
Pain over time intensifies
Hopelessness ensues, further diminishing quality of life

Treatment of myofascial pain generally requires a health care provider with a specialty in pain management.

BARRIERS TO TREATMENT

Chronic back pain is one of the greatest problems in health care, and it often goes unrecognized for the devastating impact it can have on individuals, families, and the community at large. For the individual and family, it is the cause of a significant amount of physical and psychosocial pain and suffering, with debilitating, long-lasting effects. From the perspective of community, it puts an enormous financial burden on our health care system, which leads to increased insurance premiums and health care costs. Billions of dollars are spent each year on medical bills and billions of dollars are lost in wages for clients disabled with back pain.

In recent years, new, more effective treatments for individuals with chronic back pain have been identified. However, there are significant barriers to clients receiving effective treatment (Table 8-2). Many primary care physicians have not been taught about myofascial pain and treatment, and they are not familiar with the existence and effectiveness of programs for this and other types of back or muscle pain. The problem is compounded by the fact that most primary care providers have not been taught how to treat the person in pain holistically, particularly when the pain is chronic. Medical training for chronic pain has been almost nonexistent.

Even when referrals are made, there is risk that treatment for chronic back pain will not be provided. Treatment provided by pain specialists may not be fully paid by third-party payers. Limitation of reimbursable visits is likely to occur when third-party payers perceive treatment as nonphysical in nature (ie, visits for instruction on behavioral strategies) or when treatment plans are not supported by a significant amount of research. Limited participation in treatment for chronic back pain runs the risk that the treatment will not be effective in providing relief or control of the pain.

Delays in referrals for appropriate treatment also pose barriers to the efficacy of treatment. Unrelieved severe pain changes the spine in such a way that prolongs and intensifies the pain experience.[3] Treatment late in the pain cycle is often less effective than treatment nearer the onset. Over time, pain intensifies and deconditioning ensues, further intensifying the pain experience. Clients undergoing such negative experiences often lose hope that they will obtain relief of their pain. Loss of hope can lead to depression, which also intensifies the negativity of the experience and diminishes the overall quality of clients' lives.

Case Study Revisited

Problems With Mrs. K.'s Experience With Chronic Back Pain

Mrs. K.'s experience with acute low back pain, which evolved into chronic back pain, exemplifies the significant deficits in the medical community's approach to this problem. The initial work-up (which ruled out a neurological deficit) was appropriate, as was the treatment plan for rest, anti-inflammatories, muscle relaxants, and heat. However, Mrs. K.'s continued bedrest and inactivity, with resulting "stiffness," and her fear that activity might cause neurological dysfunction indicated that she lacked knowledge about the importance of activity and the possible relationship of inactivity with stiffness. Her inactivity and stiffness likely intensified her pain and acted as a barrier to her recovery.

The absence of a full assessment of Mrs. K.'s pain experience, her release from treatment despite the presence of ongoing pain, the absence of imaging studies after 12 weeks of back pain, and the lack of recommendations or referrals for evaluation and potentially effective treatment provide further evidence that the plan of care was inadequate. Mrs. K.'s treatment did not meet the standard of care that should be provided for back pain. However, given that this treatment scenario is so common (ie, no referral to a pain specialist), it is likely that many (if not most) health care providers and third-party payers would perceive Mrs. K.'s treatment as appropriate.

Appropriate treatment for Mrs. K. should have included assessments for the impact the pain had on her physical function, level of frustration and distress, and quality of life. Mrs. K. should also have been told that true herniations of discs are not very common and that some activity or exercise would likely enhance her recovery, not put her in danger. She should have been referred to a pain specialist or at the very least a physical therapist who is experienced in back pain to assist with a structured plan of activity tailored to her individual needs. Interventions such as local ice applications and relaxation techniques would also have been appropriate. Mrs. K. may also have benefited from referral for therapeutic manipulation (adjustment) of the spine by a chiropractor or osteopath, particularly when her pain was acute. Research has shown that spinal manipulation is effective in relieving pain and improving physical function in a significant number of clients with acute low back pain.[2] Research supporting the effect of manipulation on chronic back pain is inconclusive as of this writing, but some clients may benefit from spinal adjustments even for chronic pain.

Case Study Resolved

Without physician referral, Mrs. K. seeks treatment with an osteopathic physician. This physician tells her that her pelvis and spine are out of alignment and performs an adjustment. She obtains relief from her pain for a few days at a time, but the pain reoccurs within a week or so after manipulation.

Hopeful that more can be done for her pain, Mrs. K. seeks a physician who specializes in back pain. In the phone book she finds a back clinic affiliated with a community hospital and a clinic for sports injuries. She is given an appointment, which involves history and physical examination by a physiatrist who is also a pain specialist.

The physical examination performed by the physiatrist differs in that in addition to assessing her neurological function, he assesses for sites of pain (trigger points) by applying deep pressure to the muscles in the buttocks (eg, glutei) and thigh. The physician identifies multiple trigger points in both buttocks and thighs, along with tenderness in the left lower part of the back. He tells her that she has myofascial pain syndrome and recommends that she have a course of physical therapy that includes ultrasonic massage to trigger points, manual trigger point massage, and gentle muscle stretching. He recommends that she initially see the physical therapist three times a week and that he will follow her progress closely. She has follow-up appointments with the specialist in 3 weeks, at which time he injects her trigger points with normal saline solution.

With this combination of therapies, Mrs. K.'s pain decreases, and she is started on a physical exercise program to strengthen the involved muscles and improve her flexibility and physical function. Over a period of 5 months, the pain in Mrs. K.'s back, buttocks, and thighs significantly decreases to the point that it occurs only with certain activities. One activity that aggravates the pain is the performance of pelvic tilts. Although the physical therapist does not understand why this exercise aggravates her pain, she states that it is essential to listen to each individual person's body and suggests that she no longer perform pelvic tilts. The physician also encourages Mrs. K. to perform her own trigger point therapy by applying pressure to trigger sites when pain recurs.

Through self-referral to a physician who specializes in chronic back pain, Mrs. K. not only obtains relief of the pain but also learns to control her pain when it reoccurs, possibly preventing its reoccurrence through stretching and gentle (not standard) exercises.

CHAPTER SUMMARY

General classifications and diagnoses of low back pain are based on duration of the pain (eg, acute versus chronic) and characteristics of physical exam and diagnostic findings that rule in or rule out certain diagnoses. Chronic low back pain can have a significantly negative impact on a person's quality of life. This, coupled with the fact that there are multiple barriers to effective treatment, make it imperative for health care providers to refer clients with unrelieved acute or chronic pain to specialists. Most primary care physicians are not educated or skilled in providing effective treatment for chronic pain syndromes. Therapies to help clients obtain relief from pain and gain more control over their pain should be offered to any client afflicted with chronic back pain.

REFERENCES

1. Long DM. *Contemporary Diagnosis and Management of Pain.* Newtown, Pa: Handbooks in Health Care; 1997.
2. Bigos S, Bowyer Q, Braen G, et al. *Acute Low Back Problems in Adults: Clinical Practice Guideline No. 14. AHCPR Pub No. 95-0643.* Rockville, Md: Agency for Health Care Policy and Research, Public Health Service, US Department of Health and Human Services; 1995.
3. Advise H, Crombie I, Brown J, Martin C. Diminishing returns or appropriate treatment strategy? An analysis of short-term outcomes after pain clinic treatment. *Pain.* 1997;70:203-208.

BIBLIOGRAPHY

Caudill M. *Managing Pain Before it Manages You.* New York: Guilford Press; 1995.

Travell JG, Simons DG. *Myofascial Pain and Dysfunction: The Trigger Point Manual.* Baltimore, Md: Williams & Wilkins; 1983.

Case Study Questions

1. Identify three questions that Mrs. K. (and you) might have asked the orthopedic surgeon while he was caring for this client.
2. Why do you think the orthopedic surgeon released Mrs. K. without ordering physical therapy and/or follow-up?
3. Why do you think Mrs. K's internist gave her no further recommendation for treatment of her back pain?
4. Which characteristic of Mrs. K's pain supports the diagnosis of myofascial pain?

Multiple-Choice Questions

1. Specific causes of back pain are:
   A. Diagnosed through a medical history
   B. Diagnosed by x-ray
   C. Diagnosed by neurological exam
   D. Difficult to diagnose

2. Acute low back pain most often originates:
   A. In the bony portion of the spine
   B. In discs
   C. Within muscles or ligaments
   D. Within the spinal canal

3. The majority of clients with acute low back pain:
   A. Have herniated discs
   B. Develop chronic low back pain syndrome
   C. Are incapacitated no longer than 1 to 2 weeks
   D. Require surgery

4. Most clients with acute low back pain do not have neurological deficits. Recommended treatment for these clients includes all of the following *except*:
   A. Bedrest for 1 week
   B. Anti-inflammatory drugs
   C. Analgesics
   D. Muscle relaxants

5. The hallmark of myofascial pain is:
   A. It improves with bedrest
   B. Referred numbness and tingling
   C. A decrease in motor function
   D. Trigger points in muscles

CASE STUDY ANSWERS

1. What is the significance of the pain in the buttocks (new location) 4 and 8 weeks post-injury? When Mrs. K. reported this new pain and the continued low back pain to the orthopedic surgeon, his reply was that there was "not a disc problem." Mrs. K., however, would have benefited from knowing what the new buttock pain represented. Also beneficial to find out is what the surgeon thought was causing the pain (if not a disc), what the expected outcome was likely to be, and if physical therapy or manipulation with a chiropractor might help or hurt.

2. Medical school teaching and textbooks have historically neglected the problem of muscle pain and the significance of myofascial trigger points and pain. If a physician has not been taught or does not recognize a myofascial trigger point problem, he or she will not order appropriate consult and treatment.

3. The internist likely released Mrs. K. without further recommendations because he believed he had ruled out a serious problem by CT scan and a negative neurological exam. A CT scan, however, would not show soft tissue injury, and a negative neurological exam does not address the problem of myofascial pain. The internist, like the orthopedic surgeon, probably did not have adequate knowledge of myofascial pain, and the diagnosis was not made.

4. Pain in her low back that radiates to the buttocks 8 weeks postsurgery. Myofascial pain often radiates to the hips, buttocks, groin, and upper thighs. The physiatrist's assessment of trigger points by applying deep pressure to the muscles in the buttocks (glutei) and thigh also characterized Mrs. K.'s pain as myofascial.

MULTIPLE-CHOICE ANSWERS

1. D. X-rays will show the bony anatomy of the spine, but soft tissue abnormalities are not well-visualized. History and physical examination assist in ruling in and ruling out certain abnormalities but often do not give definitive information as to the specific cause of back pain.

2. C. Most causes of acute low back pain originate within muscles or ligaments of the back.

3. C. True disc herniation is actually a rare cause of back pain. Acute back pain is self-limiting and benign, and most clients are incapacitated no longer than 1 or 2 weeks. If neurological deficits are not involved, immediate surgery for back pain is generally not necessary.

4. A. Bedrest for clients with acute back pain should be limited to 3 days or less.

5. D. Trigger points are thought to occur either primary or secondary to prolonged muscle spasm.

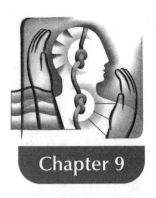

Chapter 9

Pain and Children

Case Study

Kelly N. is a 3-year-old girl who is admitted to the surgical day unit to have her tonsils and adenoids removed. She is in otherwise good health. Her mother and father accompany her. Although they have been given information by the pediatrician about what to expect, they both appear very anxious. During the admission process, EMLA cream is applied to Kelly's right forearm in preparation for intravenous access. The nurse anesthetist starts the IV with little discomfort to the client. Kelly is taken to the operating room, where surgery is completed with minimal blood loss and no complications. She is transferred to the postanesthesia care unit where she receives one dose of IV morphine for discomfort. Once she is assessed as stable, she is transferred to the pediatric unit to continue recovering from anesthesia. The plan of care is to continue pain management and hydration until it is determined that she can drink fluids and use oral pain medication. At that point, she will be discharged to home with her parents. The standard of care in this hospital for an uncomplicated tonsillectomy is discharge within 12 hours of surgery.

Pediatric clients make up a group with very special needs when it comes to pain management. Communication issues and ways these clients respond to adverse events make assessment for pain different and more challenging. The challenge of using medication safely for pain control is presented because of the differences in uptake and metabolism. Varied developmental stages require varied approaches to comfort, social support, and behavioral approaches to pain relief. Including the parents in treatment decisions can be extremely important, but at the same time attempting to not overwhelm them with information and tasks.

Pediatric clients are usually grouped according to developmental stage. Infants are usually defined as birth to 1 year of age; children, 1 year through 11 years of age; and adolescents, 12 through 18 years of age. Children may be further grouped into toddlers, pre-school-aged children, and school-aged children. All three groups have different levels of physical and psychosocial development, and differing developmental tasks. Both physical and psychosocial developmental stages should be considered when developing assessment and treatment plans for pain in the pediatric client. Elements at each stage of development affect how the pain is perceived and relief measures that will be appropriate and helpful.

> The child's stage of physical and psychosocial development directly affects pain perception, expression, and intervention.

The healthy child is more apt to experience acute forms of pain rather than chronic pain. Chronic pain is a factor in pediatric chronic illnesses or conditions and in congenital conditions. Acute pain may be the result of illness or occur with trauma, surgical intervention, or invasive diagnostic or treatment procedures. Pain in this client population is seen across treatment settings, from home to outpatient ambulatory settings, surgical and dental settings, inpatient acute care facilities, long-term care facilities, and hospice. Simple acute pain is one of the most frequent reasons for accessing pediatric care. This type of pain is often related to middle ear infection or swimmer's ear, teething pain, abdominal pain related to gastroenteritis or appendicitis, sore throat related to streptococcus infection or tonsillitis, or pain as the result of accidental trauma. The parent or adult caregiver is frequently the first one to identify the pain because of changes in the child's activity or demeanor. Depending on the changes noted and the adult's perceived severity of the pain or an assumption on the part of the adult as to the possible cause of the pain, independent measures for pain relief will be used or the child's health care provider will be called. Parents of young children who suffer frequent ear infections, for example, become expert at identifying pain-related behaviors such as changes in sleep and eating patterns, crying that is different from the norm, or self-comforting behaviors such rubbing or tugging the affected ear. Experience builds a set of assessment parameters for these parents, and attention is more rapidly paid to these behaviors as indicating pain in the child.

> Parents of young children build their own assessment criteria. A parent is very often accurate in describing his or her young child's pain.

Historically, pediatric clients have had less successful interventions for pain than adults. The reasons for this vary. The child's ability to express or communicate pain through behavior is often lacking and is sometimes unrecognized. It is important to remember that a child is not a small adult. A health care provider cannot successfully provide interventions for what cannot be comprehensively assessed. To provide more successful intervention, better assessment tools and parameters must be identified for this population. Poor assessment impacts administration of analgesics or narcotics when the medication is ordered on an as-needed (PRN) basis. Pain medication is often ordered to be given PRN, resulting in less effective pain relief for the often difficult-to-assess pediatric client. A PRN dosing schedule treats pain rather than attempts to keep the client relatively pain-free.

> The health care professional cannot intervene for that which cannot be adequately assessed.

Many health care providers are reluctant to use narcotics in the pain relief plan for pediatric clients, choosing to use less potent analgesics. Even when narcotics have been ordered, many nurses hesitate to choose them on a PRN basis, administering an ordered NSAID instead. As described in the Department of Health and Human Services pain management guidelines,[1,2] when narcotics are used the dose is usually small, potentially inadequate to relieve pain; and time between doses is long, further hindering pain relief. This may relate to a caregiver's reluctance to use narcotics or inability to effectively assess subtle cues indicating the presence of pain in the pediatric client. Adding to this problem is the current trend to order pain medication on a PRN basis. When subtle cues are missed in the assessment process, pain increases in severity before medication is offered for relief. Parents are included in the assessment process but are sometimes not believed. The first step to formulating a plan for adequate pain management in children as with all others is adequate, appropriate, and thorough assessment.

ASSESSING THE PEDIATRIC CLIENT FOR PAIN

How is it appropriate to assess the child for pain? What parameters are used? Children at different developmental stages react differently to pain. Reactions do not always seem to match severity. By being aware of useful parameters at different stages of development, the health care provider can more expertly assess and plan intervention.

Neonates (very young infants) cry as a result of pain. The intensity of the cry and associated vital signs may not indicate the intensity of the pain sensation. The cry may be weak, and heart rate and blood pressure may decrease instead of increasing.

As infants mature, crying continues to be the response to pain. Parents can often identify a distinctive cry related to pain that is different from other crying. Body movements will also change to indicate pain, including squirming, restlessness, and tugging at the painful area. Young infants will cry loudly and hold their bodies rigidly. Older infants react more specifically to pain, attempting to push away a painful stimulus. At this developmental point, heart rate and blood

> Many parents of infants and toddlers can describe hearing a characteristic cry in the night and awaken to finding their child tugging at one ear. "Aha!" they think, "Another ear infection."

pressure are commonly elevated with pain. The older infant with a history of pain, especially painful procedures, may withdraw. Assessment in infants should include behavioral signs, like crying, and more subtle signs of pain, including body postures and vital signs.

Toddlers are more readily able to begin to engage in verbal communication but are still unable to talk about their pain. Physiological response to pain is similar to that of infants—loud, lusty crying and physical efforts to avoid painful stimulus. Toddlers in pain can be restless, even appearing hyperactive, even when increased activity exacerbates pain. This occurs because the toddler does not cognitively associate increased activity with increased pain. It is very important to be aware of this fact, because many adult caregivers tend to associate increasing levels of activity with feeling better. This is not necessarily so with the toddler. Expressions of pain continue to vary at this stage and with varied and emerging personality traits of each individual child, as well as increasing ability to communicate verbally.

Preschool-aged children are more developed in their verbal abilities, perceive the world in a very concrete and fixed way, have grave concerns about bodily mutilation, and can engage in magical thinking. These factors make assessment for pain very different from the younger child. Enhanced verbal abilities allow the preschooler to describe location and intensity of pain. Simple assessment scales are useful at this age, but scales involving numbers or printed words can be confusing or distracting. Intensity of color on a linear chart may be useful or the common happy to sad faces assessment tool (see Figure 2-5).

Verbal description scales such as "no pain, a little pain, a lot of pain, the worst pain" can be useful in evaluation of treatment, but it is important to keep the wording consistent. The preschool-aged child's reaction to pain may seem out of proportion with the event or the child's description of the pain. Fears, magical thinking, or a sense of self-blame may complicate this reaction. This child may also lash out angrily at caregivers, especially those involved in invasive procedures.

School-aged children have much improved powers of communication. They learn quickly, assimilating information, but giving it their own individual meaning. Thinking is very concrete. At this stage, the child can verbally describe location, intensity, and type or characteristics of pain, and can use most pain assessment scales. Avoid the temptation to treat this age group as a small adult. They are more passive than younger children about accepting pain and are much less able to verbalize requests for assistance or relief than the adult client.

Adolescents are even more developed in their ability to communicate but are frequently reluctant to communicate. Although they are well able to use assessment tools, their reluctance in communication requires the health care provider to assess for more subtle signs of pain. These include psychosocial withdrawal, decreased levels of activity, increased anger, suspicion or anxiety, or increased complaints about issues unrelated to pain. Vital signs such as blood pressure and heart rate generally increase with pain in this age group. Issues with sexuality and developing body image add to the adolescent's reluctance to express pain.

It is not at all uncommon for a pediatric client to regress to thinking and behaviors that express pain to a younger developmental age group. The school-aged child may act more like a preschooler or even a toddler. The toddler may only cry, not using developed verbal skills at all. Children who have recently achieved a developmental milestone, such as sentence construction or toilet training, may revert to old habits in the presence of pain. The preceding descriptions are useful as cues to assessment, but each individual pediatric client must be approached with assessment techniques that are appropriate for that individual.

Pain Management Strategies for the Pediatric Client

Strategies for pain control in this age group include pharmacological, physical, and behavioral options. All three options must be tailored to the age and developmental level of the child.

Children use and metabolize medications in very different ways than adults. The safe and routine pediatric doses of medications are different from those of adults. It is the responsibility of the health care professional ordering or administering medication to be aware of these dose parameters, which are readily available from package inserts or drug reference books, including the hospital formulary.

NSAIDs, acetaminophen, and salicylates like aspirin are appropriate for use in this client population, with adjustment for the correct dose. These are useful for mild to moderate pain and will also help with fever reduction. An NSAID or acetaminophen would be a more appropriate choice. This vital information should be shared with all parents of small children.

> Never use aspirin for children with viral symptoms, flu-like symptoms, or fever because of the risk of developing Reye's syndrome.

In the case of more severe pain or after procedures in which severe pain can be expected, opioids are a safe and effective medication choice to use in children. As with all clients receiving opioids, careful monitoring for side effects, excessive sedation, or respiratory depression is necessary. Positioning the very small or sedated child to maintain a patent airway is an important consideration. Treating for unpleasant side effects such as nausea and vomiting is also essential in this age group. As with adults, including an NSAID in the medication profile when possible can increase pain relief or prevention and may reduce the amount of opioid necessary.

Adjuvant medications to potential opioid use to promote relaxation, sedation, or reduce side effects are a third medication type to include in the plan of care. Local anesthetics, such as EMLA cream, are good choices to prevent procedural-related pain.

> An important goal in pain management for children is prevention instead of relief for pain that has already occurred.

Routes of administration depend on a wide variety of factors in this population. Oral administration is appropriate when the child can safely swallow, when there is no need for rapid titration, and when oral intake is allowed. One other factor when choosing oral administration is the level of cooperation offered by the client. Children who resist oral medication and make it a continual battle to provide medication may require another administration route.

Rectal administration is possible and a good choice for neonates and infants. Toddlers may react negatively, perceiving this route as very invasive and confusing at a time when toilet training is in progress. Older age groups may also perceive it as invasive because of boundary, developmental, and sexuality issues.

> At times, it is necessary to cut a suppository in half to administer the required dose. Most suppositories should be split down the middle the long way, because medication is usually dispersed in the back of the tablet, with the head being glycerin or another inert material. Unfortunately, this leaves a long sliver that may be difficult to insert without breaking. A few extra minutes of refrigeration may make it easier to handle. Don't forget to share this information with parents who may have to give their children suppositories at home.

Subcutaneous or intramuscular injections are also administration choices in children, but because they are also a cause of pain, they should be chosen only when absolutely necessary, especially with children younger than school age.

Intravenous administration is a good alternative when rapid titration of medication is necessary or when other routes are unacceptable. Use of a local anesthetic prior to intravenous insertion is desirable for this population. The IV site must be well protected in younger children who do not understand its purpose or cannot be reasoned with or instructed not to tug at it. Neonates and infants are often difficult to achieve peripheral intravenous lines on, because of large amounts of subcutaneous fat in the arms and legs. One alternative is use of a superficial scalp vein, but this can be very distressing to mom or dad.

Less invasive alternatives, such as administration across a mucous membrane, are becoming popular when caring for children. One excellent example is the fentanyl oralet (transmucosal fentanyl citrate), which is used to induce conscious sedation prior to procedures like closed reduction of a fracture. The narcotic analgesic is supplied as a flavored lozenge and mounted on a handle like a lollipop. When the child sucks on the lozenge, the fentanyl citrate is absorbed through the mucosal tissues and gastrointestinal tract.

Patient-controlled analgesia (PCA) pumps are useful in older school-aged children and adolescents. They are especially effective in these two groups by allowing the real sense of control over pain relief. They are also very useful for adolescents who are not willing to verbalize pain needs. A PCA pump is not useful in younger children who cannot learn its use and should not be an alternative for parents to administer IV medication.

Case Study Revisited

Kelly becomes very restless, frequently crying and clinging to her mother within an hour of returning to the pediatric unit. She rubs at her throat and drools, seeming reluctant to swallow. Her mom requests some pain medication for her. Although IV morphine has been ordered, there is also an order for Tylenol PO or rectally administered. The nurse chooses Tylenol suspension, which Kelly is very reluctant to swallow. Much of it ends up on Kelly's pajamas. Soon after receiving the medication, Kelly vomits. She continues to cry and refuses to drink or even suck on ice chips. Her only source of hydration is intravenous fluid.

After 2½ hours of crying and restless behavior, her mother requests "anything" to relieve Kelly's discomfort. When the nurse appears with more Tylenol suspension, Kelly refuses to swallow it, screaming. Her mother thinks a suppository is "a really bad idea for Kelly." Mom is frustrated and angry. Unsure what to do next, the nurse calls the clinical nurse specialist (CNS) for help.

The CNS explains the safety and efficacy of using opioids in children. She administers one dose to Kelly and helps her mom place an ice pack at her throat. It is not until her second dose 2 hours later that she begins to settle down and act like a comfortable child. Once she is comfortable, she takes some bites of an ice pop and later agrees to drink. In her discussion with the staff nurse, the CNS explains that pain relief and hydration are two important goals for clients like Kelly. Dehydration frequently exacerbates nausea and vomiting.

PHYSICAL STRATEGIES FOR PAIN MANAGEMENT IN CHILDREN

Physical strategies for this client population include the use of touch, massage, and physical contact; application of heat and cold; changes in position; and activity or exercise. Infants and toddlers crave contact with their mothers. Having mom able to hold or snuggle the baby helps in providing comfort, security, and trust, and promotes reduction of tension. Gentle, rhythmic stroking and superficial massage is useful in all pediatric stages, however permission and explanations are necessary with older school-aged children and adolescents who have a strong sense of privacy about their bodies. Deep massage should only be used when there is no risk of bleeding or embolization.

BEHAVIORAL APPROACHES TO PAIN MANAGEMENT IN CHILDREN

Behavioral strategies in the pediatric client depend heavily on the developmental stage of the client. Neonates and infants are egocentric, with presence of a mother figure as a source of comfort. Allowing the infant to be held even during an invasive procedure increases the sense of comfort. A quiet environment and soft verbal stimulation such as singing or humming can provide distraction and soothe an anxious or crying infant. Toddlers also respond to this approach, but when they become overly active as a response to pain, holding them seems restrictive, resulting in further increases in activity. Although toddlers are beginning to verbalize, they can comprehend only the most basic instruction. Don't try to reason with a toddler. Give quiet verbal commands, and keep the environment quiet and nonthreatening.

> Never try reasoning with a toddler!

Invasive procedures for all age groups in the pediatric population should be done in a specific place, especially away from the bedside in an inpatient facility, to provide a safe place.

Preschool-aged children are more responsive to words and actions that take into account their sense of magical thinking. Because this age group has fear of mutilation and is just beginning to establish body image boundaries, invasive procedures are anxiety provoking. A well-placed bandage after any invasive procedure or injury, no matter how small, will prevent leaks, maintain body integrity, and provide a concrete notice of the event. Behavioral approaches with preschoolers should also be aimed very simply at helping the child to understand that he or she is not to blame for an illness or trauma.

School-aged children and adolescents need to maintain a sense of control and privacy. Giving them *realistic* choices concerning treatment, timing, and perhaps route of administration may result in greater compliance with a plan of care. This age group should definitely be included in designing their own plan of care. They are capable of learning many of the behavioral approaches to pain management that are useful in the adult population. It is very important to remember that they are in the process of achieving very different and important developmental tasks and should not be treated like an adult. School-aged children are excellent gatherers of information and are sensitive to truth telling. It is important to be honest and retain their trust. They and adolescents have already begun to establish individual coping behaviors. They should be encouraged to use familiar coping strategies.

Managing pain in the pediatric client is an interactive process involving health care professionals, parents, and children. When caring for the family as a unit, it is important to remember not to overwhelm a parent with tasks or responsibilities. For a parent, seeing his or her child in pain is a significantly stressful event. Trust and information provided by the health care professional will help to mediate some of that stress. Feelings of helplessness or failure make it worse. When identifying the plan of care, consider the parent along with the child. Set goals that are mutually agreeable and maintain a dialogue. Successful pain management occurs with successful interaction.

Case Study Resolved

After a third dose of morphine on the pediatric unit, Kelly began drinking in amounts adequate for hydration. Before removing her IV though, the nurse wants to be certain that oral pain medication will be adequate to relieve pain. Kelly adamantly refuses, in true 3-year old fashion, to take the Tylenol suspension when it is offered, but she will chew and swallow chewable tablets. Confident that her pain is well relieved after a second dose of Tylenol and since there have been no more episodes of vomiting, the nurse removes the IV and prepares Kelly for discharge.

REFERENCES

1. Acute Pain Management Guideline Panel. Acute pain management in infants, children, and adolescents: operative procedures. *Quick Reference Guide for Clinicians. No. 1a. AHCPR Pub No. 92-0019.* Rockville, Md: Agency for Health Care Policy and Research, Public Health Service, US Department of Health and Human Services; 1992.
2. Acute Pain Management Guideline Panel. *Acute Pain Management: Operative or Medical Procedures and Trauma. AHCPR Pub No. 92-0032.* Rockville, Md: Agency for Health Care Policy and Research, Public Health Service, US Department of Health and Human Services; 1992.

BIBLIOGRAPHY

Karch AM. *2002 Lippincott's Nursing Drug Guide.* Philadelphia, Pa: Lippincott; 2001.

McCaffery M, Pasero C. *Pain: Clinical Manual.* St. Louis, Mo: Mosby; 1999.

Wong DL. *Waley & Wong's Essentials of Pediatric Nursing.* 5th ed. St. Louis, Mo: Mosby; 1998.

Wong DL, Perry SE. *Maternal Child Nursing Care.* St. Louis, Mo: Mosby; 1998.

World Health Organization. *Cancer Pain Relief and Palliative Care in Children.* Geneva, Switzerland: Author; 1998.

Yaster M, Krane EJ, Kaplan RF, et al. *Pediatric Pain Management and Sedation Handbook.* St. Louis, Mo: Mosby; 1997.

MULTIPLE-CHOICE QUESTIONS

1. Which of the following is true regarding pain in children?
   A. Children have poorly developed nociceptors, so they do not frequently experience severe pain
   B. Pain management in children is similar to management in adults
   C. Pain management in children is frequently more challenging than in adults
   D. Children metabolize medications more quickly than adults

2. Which assessment parameter is essential in evaluating a pediatric client for pain management?
   A. Height and weight
   B. Developmental stage
   C. Social support
   D. All of the above

3. Behaviors used to express pain in children:
   A. Always involve regression in developmental stage
   B. Frequently seem unrelated to the source of pain
   C. Do not differ from behaviors seen in adults
   D. Are unreliable and should not be considered as part of pain assessment

4. Acute pain in children:
   A. Is always the result of trauma
   B. May be related to illness, intervention, or trauma
   C. Is less commonly seen than chronic pain
   D. Is seen only in specific health care settings

5. Use of medication administered on a PRN or as-needed basis for children with pain:
   A. Frequently results in poor pain management because of inappropriate assessment
   B. Is restricted to use only in critical care settings
   C. Provides excellent pain management
   D. Is never used as an alternative in planning that client's care

6. The first step in designing a plan for pain management in pediatric clients is:
   A. Height and weight
   B. Interview with parents, grandparents, and siblings
   C. Offering distraction and play therapy
   D. A complete and thorough assessment

7. Preschool children, although often able to verbalize their pain, frequently do not report it accurately as a result of all of the following except:
   A. Fear
   B. Magical thinking
   C. Concerns about bodily mutilation
   D. Lack of maternal trust

8. Safe and routine pediatric doses of medication are:
   A. Always half of the appropriate adult dose
   B. Specific to each medication
   C. Never shared with parents
   D. Found on the label of unit-dosed packages

9. Use of narcotic medications with small children may result in sedation. The *most important* nursing intervention for these small clients is to:
   A. Position the child to maintain a patent airway
   B. Not use adjunct medications to treat unpleasant side effects
   C. Caution against operating heavy machinery
   D. Reduce the dose of medication until sedation is no longer apparent

10. Rectal administration of medication is frequently most appropriate in which age group?
    A. Infants
    B. Toddlers
    C. Preschool-aged children
    D. Adolescents

MULTIPLE-CHOICE ANSWERS

1. C
2. D
3. B
4. B
5. A
6. D
7. D
8. B
9. A
10. A

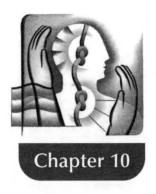

Chapter 10

Pain and the Elderly

Case Study

Mrs. G., an 87-year-old woman who lives in a nursing home, is referred to the nurse practitioner during sick call. Mrs. G. is suffering from early-stage Alzheimer's disease. She has been complaining to the nurses of right-sided abdominal pain and flank pain for 2 days. They have observed her rubbing or holding her right side as well. She is afebrile and denies nausea or changes in bowel routine. Her appetite is somewhat diminished. Upon examination, her upper right quadrant is tender to touch, but no guarding or abdominal rigidity is noted. She has bowel sounds in all four quadrants.

The growth of the elderly as a segment of the national population challenges health care providers to respond to their specific issues. Factors encouraging the growth of the elderly population include the graying of the baby boomers, extension of the life span, improvements in screening for and treatment of disease, and economic shifts. Some specific needs of this population stem from their higher predisposition to illness, both chronic and acute, as well as higher rates of terminal illnesses. Related to their increased health care needs is the problem of pain in the elderly population, which is a frequent occurrence with multiple chronic as well as acute conditions. Assessment is vitally important to attempt to identify the source and type of pain, especially with the complication of multiple problems that the elderly client may experience. Confusion or dementia, hearing or vision loss, or isolation may further confuse assessment attempts.

There is no reason to believe that the elderly client does not experience pain or that the pain experience is reduced with aging. No normal physiological changes associated with aging are responsible for diminishing pain sensations. The elderly do experience changes in the natural aging process, which put them at higher risk for injury and illness with related pain, as well as changes that may interfere with attempts at interventions for pain relief. By specifically targeting assessment and intervention techniques to the individual elderly client in pain, successful pain relief is a possibility.

What causes pain in the elderly client? The causes are as varied as the clients themselves. Pain may be an acute phenomenon associated with trauma, injury, illness, or surgery. Age-related changes in visual acuity, hearing, mobility, balance, and judgment increase the elder client's propensity for accidents and traumatic injury. Loss in body mass—muscular, fatty, or subcutaneous tissue—results in the potential for greater injury than for younger clients in the same traumatic instance. Osteoporosis, a loss of bone density, results in the potential for fractures. Subcutaneous tissue loss often results in fine, tissue paper-thin skin that is easily torn. Even slight dehydration causes changes in skin turgor, which can result in easier or more extensive injury. Injuries to the skin, subcutaneous tissues, muscles, tendons, ligaments, or bones may result in an inflammatory response, mediated by the immune system. Breaks in the skin or mucous membranes are potential avenues for the development of infection. Infections also result in immune and inflammatory responses. Chemical mediators of the inflammatory response are also chemical mediators in the pain process, so elders at risk for these problems are at increased risk for pain. Normal changes in the aging process *do not* involve a breakdown or weakening of the immune system, so inflammation continues to be a natural response to injury in the elderly client.

> Multiple physical changes occur with aging. They may be a part of the natural aging process or may be related to illness or trauma. It is important to consider these changes when planning interventions.

Manifestation of pain may occur or change with vascular changes associated with aging. Anginal pain or intermittent claudication may accompany arterial insufficiency related to atherosclerosis or hypertension. Peripheral neuropathies may reduce or completely inhibit the sensation of pain in the affected extremities, thus restricting the protective mechanisms associated with pain. Neuropathies are frequently associated with venous changes, diabetes mellitus, or use of certain neurotoxic medications. Peripheral neuropathies are generally not reversible. Pain sensation may be masked by the use of prescribed or over-the-counter medication. Many elderly clients use pain medication for chronic conditions such as osteoarthritis. Even the use of aspirin as a cardioprotective may reduce the pain response. For this reason, it is very important to document a comprehensive medication history when assessing an elderly client for pain.

Frequent interface with the health care professional is yet another reason for the experience of pain for the elderly client. Painful diagnostic procedures, surgical procedures, treatments, and rehabilitation all account for instances of iatrogenic pain. Prior to certain invasive procedures, medications used for the treatment of chronic pain that interfere with blood clotting, such as NSAIDs or aspirin, must be curtailed. It is important to identify alternate pain relief interventions appropriate for the client to use in the absence of his or her usual relief measures.

Multiple medical conditions that occur more commonly as the client ages are related to increased incidences of pain. Chronic conditions,

> Alternate relief measures for pain in the elderly client include:
>
> | | |
> |---|---|
> | Relaxation | Distraction |
> | Heat therapy | Cold therapy |
> | Exercise | Change in position |
> | Massage | |

including osteoarthritis, result in pain that may significantly affect the elderly client's quality of life and is responsible for self-medication as well as increased visits to the doctor or nurse practitioner. Cancers are more common in the elderly client as well. With improvements in treatment and detection of many types of cancer, the associated pain is often in the chronic phase of the illness.

> Pain from cancer is usually a late occurrence; it is rarely an early indicator of the disease.

Pre-existing or chronic illnesses may mask manifestations of acute pain or delay appropriate intervention for acute pain.

Changes in mental status commonly associated with aging, including senescence or Alzheimer's disease, complicate manifestation of acute and chronic pain. The client may not vocalize pain or may act in ways frequently associated with pain. Alternate and client-specific assessment strategies must be used for these clients to determine the presence of pain and the success of interventions.

Physiological Changes of Aging

Normal and illness-related physiological changes exist in the elderly client who is experiencing pain. These changes must be considered in assessment and intervention strategies, especially when using pharmacological interventions.

> Routes of medication administration include:
>
> | | |
> |---|---|
> | Oral | Transbuccal |
> | Through G-tube or J-tube | Rectal |
> | Transcutaneous | Subcutaneous |
> | Intramuscular | Intravenous |

Routes of administration should be carefully considered in relation to age-related changes. Oral routes can be affected by changes in swallowing ability, changes in the amount of oral secretions, and changes in digestion. Carefully assess the client's ability to swallow tablets. If swallowing is a problem, consider breaking the tablet into smaller pieces or crushing it to administer it with thickened liquids such as applesauce or dissolved in water or juice. Tablets that are designed for timed release or with enteric coatings should not be broken or crushed. Many medications are available in liquid or suspension forms as an alternative to tablets. To assist the client in swallowing tablets, have him or her sit upright if possible. Place the tablet at the front of the tongue for better control. If the tablet is placed at the back of the mouth, it is sometimes more difficult to swallow. Swallowing is easier with only one tablet at a time. Clients who take multiple medications at one time often attempt to swallow them all at once. This practice could result in aspiration or choking for the client who has difficulty swallowing. After administering pills to an elderly client, examine the mouth to assure they have been swallowed. This could prevent choking later, in addition to making certain that the medicine will not be found on the floor or in the bed clothes later. Clients who are dehydrated or complain of a dry mouth (such as elderly clients on antihypertensive medications or diuretics) may complain of difficulty swallowing pills because they "stick" to the oral mucosa. A small sip of juice or water prior to giving the client pills frequently helps with this complaint. Clients with hiatal hernias or acid reflux often complain that pills cause an increase in discomfort. Reduced stomach motility may interfere with timely absorption of medication taken orally.

Transbuccal administration, medication absorbed across the buccal membrane (mucous membranes under the tongue or between the gums and cheek), can be problematic because of dry mouth, fragile membranes, dentures, or poor circulation. Clients with a dry mouth, which may occur as a natural change in aging or from medications or medical conditions, may experience difficulty with medications administered via this route. Insufficient moisture may slow or prevent the tablet from dissolving. The tablets may become stuck or may damage already fragile mucous membranes. Damage to the oral mucous membranes will result in pain and inflammation. Inflammation will interfere with transbuccal absorption. Dental appliances may get in the way of tablet placement. Tablets may also become caught under dentures, causing injury. Some medications are now available as sprays for transbuccal administration. Finally, in the elderly client with swallowing difficulties and/or mentation changes, placement of pills under the tongue or between the gum and cheek may present an aspiration hazard.

Transcutaneous absorption of medication may be affected by metabolism, skin or subcutaneous tissue, or by circulation. Many medications can be administered using this route, including nitropaste and fentanyl. Clients who are febrile will absorb and metabolize medication across the skin more quickly. This results in poor pain relief prior to the next administration. Loss of subcutaneous tissue or poor peripheral circulation causes poor absorption and movement of the medication into circulation. When placing transdermal medication on elderly clients, attempt to choose a spot on the trunk, avoiding the limbs. Monitor the client for fever. Assess the area of placement for pallor or mottling, signs of poor circulation. Avoid scarred areas or open areas such as skin tears or abrasions. Patches with adhesives or tape to hold patches in place should be used and removed with caution, as elderly clients' skin may be fragile and easily torn.

Subcutaneous injection is an option that has similar drawbacks for use in the elder population. Loss of subcutaneous tissue reduces areas for the medication to deposit. Changes in peripheral circulation may reduce transport of the medication into systemic circulation, reducing effective pain control. Careful assessment of the injection site for symptoms of circulatory compromise, including atrophy, pallor, and mottling, will reduce some of the transport problems. Choosing a site for injection on the trunk, especially the abdomen (avoiding the umbilicus or any areas of varicosity), is also beneficial to better pain control. Some specific advantages to using subcutaneous injection include the fact that the needle is small and fine, making a relatively painless injection technique. Bruising or bleeding are infrequent complications. This form of administering is a technique that can readily be taught to clients and their families.

Intramuscular injection is problematic in the elderly client who has lost muscle tissue to atrophy, wasting, or loss of body mass. Careful choice of site should consider the volume of medication to be injected, as decreased muscle mass reduces the area for storage or deposit of medication. Atrophy caused by circulatory insufficiencies is a good indicator that transport of the injected medication to central circulation will be poor. Finally, intramuscular injections may be extremely painful, especially when administered to a muscle that is not in a state of relaxation. Proper positioning and relaxation techniques are good aids to preventing muscle tension.

Rectal administration is often a good choice when the oral route is not a possibility for reasons such as nausea and vomiting or difficulty swallowing. Some particular considerations when using this route for the elderly client include comfort, safety, bowel habits, and cardiac history. Suppositories are made up of inert solid material that melts, such as glycerin, allowing the medication to be absorbed across the rectal mucosa. The suppository must be retained in the rectal vault long enough for melting and absorption. Clients suffering from diarrhea or rectal irritation may not be able to tolerate resisting the urge to defecate, thus expelling the suppository before the medication is absorbed. Clients with hemorrhoids often complain of intense discomfort when suppositories are inserted. Elderly clients may have difficulty lying in a position to facilitate insertion. Using the rectal route for self-administration of pain medication is repellent to some clients. In addition, stimulation of the vasovagal response when medication is inserted rectally is potentially dangerous to clients with a cardiac history. Even absent of a history of cardiac problems, vagal stimulation may result in a drop in cardiac rate and blood pressure, resulting in syncope. Assess the elderly client carefully before using this route and provide safety measures including protection from falls and other consequences of syncope, as well as ready access to a bathroom, commode, or bedpan should the rectal insertion stimulate a strong urge for a bowel movement. It is important to know that colostomy stomas can be used for insertion of rectal medication. Absorption across the mucous membranes of ileostomy or urinary diversion stomas is less certain, primarily because of the consistent nature of the drainage.

Intravenous access allows for medication to be administered directly into the circulatory system. It allows for rapid pain relief, but the medication is not stored, resulting in relief of a shorter duration. Intravenous access in elderly clients can be difficult because of poor peripheral circulation, dehydration, or noncompliance. A central line is a possibility in these cases but is more difficult to care for (especially out of the acute care environment), has the potential for complications such as hemorrhage or infection, and is more difficult and painful to insert.

In addition to physical changes that affect the choice of routes of administration, changes that affect the metabolism or storage of medication within the body occur as a part of aging. Age-related changes in the liver could affect the biotransformation of certain medications. Biotransformation refers to the conversion of medications to chemical states, which are more bioavailable for use within the body. Transformation time increases, resulting in longer elevated serum levels of drugs. Dosage intervals should be increased and maximum doses should be carefully adhered to, preventing damage to the liver from accumulation of drugs or drug metabolites. Acetaminophen is one excellent example of a drug, which is widely used by this population for pain control and is transformed in the liver.

Age-related changes within the kidneys affect renal clearance and excretion of drugs and drug metabolites, also resulting in longer periods of optimal or elevated serum drug levels. These changes may be obvious as signs and symptoms of mild, moderate, or severe renal failure or can be occult. Dehydration exacerbates this phenomenon. Decreasing the dose and increasing dose intervals will accommodate this change. It is very important to assess the client frequently, not only for adequate pain relief but also for signs and symptoms related to expected side effects and toxicity. Morphine sulfate is a good example of a frequently used medication for pain that is cleared through the kidneys.

Normal or expected physiological changes in the elderly client do not include an expected decrease in immunity; however, this is a problem experienced by many elderly clients. A decrease in effective function of the immune system can be related to many factors. Malnutrition or a decrease in intake of food and fluids as well as various disease processes has been implicated in immunocompromise. Use of medications as treatment for various comorbidities may cause a reduction in function of the elder client's immune response. Some of these medications include antineoplastics, cardiac medications, steroids, other hormone replacements, and the use of antibiotics. Reduced immune response should be evaluated and considered when selecting interventions for pain as well as administration alternatives. Use of narcotics or other interventions that may reduce mobility in the immunocompromised client carry the potential for complications of immobility such as pneumonia or skin breakdown.

The elderly client frequently exhibits alterations in mobility. Immobility or other potential complications can be exacerbated or related to medications used for pain relief, or even to nonpharmacological interventions for pain. These complications include skin breakdown, constipation, urinary tract infection, deep vein thrombosis (DVT) and embolization, pneumonia, problems with digestion and respiration, isolation, and depression. Use of sedating medication such as opioids may decrease a client's already compromised mobility. Opioids can cause or exacerbate constipation and nausea. They may depress respiration. Use of NSAIDs can cause bleeding dyscrasias or be difficult to use with anticoagulants for treating deep vein thromboses. Changes in mobility may reduce positioning or activity options as nonpharmacological interventions. By assessing the client's mobility and potential for problems initially and throughout the period that pain relief interventions are used, complications can be prevented or treated and resolved at early stages. One example is bowel status. Assessment of the client's baseline or premorbid bowel habits provides target criteria for comfort while using opioids. Increasing dietary fiber and fluid intake, and using a bulk laxative and stool softener as a bowel regimen will prevent constipation and impaction as complications of immobility and medication side effects. Continued assessment for the efficacy of both pain relief and bowel regiment with changes in the plan of care as appropriate are necessary throughout the intervention period.

Changes in mentation, including confusion, anxiety, and depression occur in the elderly, complicating both assessment for discomfort as well as alternatives for pain management. These changes will be addressed later in this chapter.

Case Study Revisited

Although Mrs. G. can indicate the location of her pain, she is unable to describe its quality. Because of this, it is two more days before a definite diagnosis of shingles is made. At this point, the characteristic rash appears. A client who does not have the complication of early Alzheimer's may have more easily been able to describe the neuroleptic nature of the pain: burning and tingling along the path of a nerve.

At this point, a mild narcotic, codeine, is prescribed along with acetaminophen and a fiber laxative nightly. Antiviral therapy is also instituted. The sedation associated with the narcotic exacerbates Mrs. G.'s confusion, and the nurses have trouble assessing her level of pain and the efficacy or pain relief methods. Mrs. G. refuses to swallow any pills, so alternate methods of administration are considered. Her antiviral medication is given intravenously, but Mrs. G. is forced to wear soft wrist restraints so she will not pull at her intravenous line. Pain medications are given subcutaneously until she is less confused and more cooperative in swallowing medications.

MEDICATION STRATEGIES

Choosing and administering medications as interventions for pain in the elderly client is complicated by many of the physiological changes that accompany aging or the comorbidities frequently seen in this population. A wide variety of medication classes are available for use in these clients with minimal restrictions. When managing acute pain, it is important to attempt to identify the source or cause of the pain and treat it, if possible. Acute pain may occur in the elderly population more frequently in addition to chronic pain syndromes. Each type of pain should be considered carefully so that appropriate treatment can be used. Medications used for one type or source of pain may not be effective for another source or type. When identifying appropriate medications, the step approach described by the clinical practice guidelines should be used. NSAIDs or salicylates are good alternatives for mild to moderate pain, with the *addition* of opioids as an alternative for more severe or unrelieved pain. Disease-specific medications for pain management should also be included in the plan of care. However, a complete medication use history is essential when planning for pharmacological intervention for pain in the elderly client. Multiple comorbidities may exist and the elder may take multiple medications, enhancing the potential for medication interactions. When taking a medication history, remember to include medications prescribed by a physician or nurse practitioner as well as self-medication. These self-prescribed medications may include symptom management with over-the-counter preparations for pain, constipation, heartburn, or a multitude of other symptoms. It may also include prescription medications that do not belong to this client. Recreational drugs should also be included in this profile. It is an unwise assumption that because the client is "old," he or she is exempt from using recreational or illicit drugs. All drugs and medications used can contribute to the problem of medication interactions. Some complications seen in the elderly population when medication interactions occur can include respiratory distress, dizziness, syncope, fatigue, sedation, constipation, dehydration, changes in blood pressure or cardiac output, changes in serum drug levels, and cardiac symptoms. Medication interactions can be mildly problematic or life-threatening. The elder population has the most potential risk for medication interactions.

Care should also be taken when choosing a medication regimen for pain relief to avoid use of medications that may complicate or mimic some of the age-related changes. Previously, the effect of medications on mobility has been discussed. Many elderly clients who use narcotics, especially morphine, as a choice for pain management express dissatisfaction with sedation, drowsiness, and depression. Depression is not a side effect of opioids, but it can be a significant symptom of pain, especially chronic pain. If the client suffers from symptoms of depression, strategies to treat the depression should be part of the plan of care. Clients who doze or nap when alone in a quiet room but are easily awakened and engaged by company or activity are not overly sedated by their pain medication. Frequently, clients who have suffered sleep deprivation because of their pain, illness, or hospitalization will sleep for long periods once their pain has been relieved. This is not medication-induced sedation. Generally, in this case, the prolonged periods of sleeping will be reduced in 24 to 48 hours. If sedation is unacceptable to the client, attempt to decrease the dose of medication and/or increase the dosage interval. Carefully assess for pain relief while manipulating the dose of medication. If a change in type or classification of medication is necessary to alleviate sedation or other side effects, use an equianalgesic table or formula to ensure adequate medication.

Side effects that occur from medications that are providing adequate pain relief can be treated independently, rather than changing an already effective medication. Some side effects about which the elderly frequently complain in addition to sedation are lightheadedness or dizziness, gastrointestinal problems, and itching. Clients using opioids, anesthetic agents, cardiac medications, and neuroleptics may report feelings of lightheadedness or a drop in blood pressure. Carefully assess the client for adequate hydration, as these symptoms can be related to or made worse by even moderate dehydration. Client teaching regarding safety is important when experiencing these symptoms.

When using NSAIDs or aspirin, clients may report heartburn, abdominal pain, or reflux. Counsel the client not to take these medications on an empty stomach, as this increases the symptoms. Use of an antacid may be of some help. Assess that overdose is not a problem. Some medications are available with an enteric coating to protect the stomach (remember, these cannot be crushed or broken for administration). Be alert for signs and symptoms of gastric ulcers or gastrointestinal bleeding. Clients using these classes of medication may also complain of nausea, which may be relieved by a bland diet and not taking the medications when the stomach is empty. Nausea and sometimes vomiting is more frequently associated with the use of narcotics, especially morphine. This can be managed with the use of a variety of antiemetics. Nausea is frequently a problem with these medications when oral intake is poor, especially when the medications are being administered orally. Codeine is a particular culprit in causing nausea. If antiemetic therapy is not appropriate or unsuccessful, then a change in medication or medication class should be considered. Constipation is another side effect associated with opioid use, which can be a problem for the elderly client. This has been discussed earlier in this chapter.

Itching with or without an accompanying rash is another frequent complaint from elders on many different types of pain medication. Although itching can sometimes be the first symptom in an anaphylactic response, usually accompanied by hives, it is normally an uncomfortable but not unsafe side effect. It can be managed with use of an antihistamine topically or systematically.

Elderly clients more frequently experience side effects from pain relief medications. This is often a consequence of age-related changes, specifically renal or hepatic changes. Reducing the dose or increasing the dosage interval may offer relief from the side effects while maintaining adequate pain control. Client teaching regarding side effects and their management are essential in helping our elderly clients comply with the pain medication regimen.

NONPHARMACOLOGICAL OPTIONS FOR PAIN CONTROL IN ELDERS

Choosing methods of pain relief in addition to (adjunct) or instead of medication has become more and more popular in recent times. When identifying alternative interventions for pain, safety, acceptability to the client, and potential for a positive outcome must be considered. Practicing holistic client-centered care and a move away from the medical model are stimuli to explore alternatives in pain management. A wide variety is available, which may be received with varied degrees of enthusiasm from the elderly client. This client population has been treated for many years utilizing the medical model. They have experienced or been aware of multiple advances in medicine and health care science. If the client does not believe that an intervention will be successful, the chances of success are seriously diminished. With this in mind, presentation of nonpharmacological methods must be positive and professional. Establishment of a therapeutic presence or therapeutic relationship is valuable in utilizing nonpharmacological methods and may be a potent intervention for relief of pain as well. The therapeutic relationship helps in relieving anxiety, muscle tension, and stress. It assists the client to a more receptive state, making client teaching, relaxation, and guided imagery easier.

Cutaneous stimulation and the use of heat and cold are alternatives for pain relief that are familiar and successful to many elderly clients. Cutaneous stimulation includes light or deep massage. Massage can be at the site of pain or in another area of the body.

Massage becomes a dangerous alternative if potential damage can be done, as when embolization is a threat. Use of heat or cold may work by utilizing the gate control theory or may be useful in reducing inflammation, thereby reducing pain. Use of heat in areas of vascular insufficiency is contraindicated. Another particular danger when using heat as pain management in this population is the risk of burns. The elderly client may be unaware of extreme temperature because of peripheral neuropathies. Skin is more fragile, frequently with diminished protective subcutaneous fat. Hot compresses should be tested by another individual for appropriate temperature, and the elderly client should avoid unsupervised use of electronic heating pads.

Distraction, relaxation, and positive use of leisure time are all realistic options, especially in adjunct pain management. Providing the elderly client with control over pain management will also enhance results. Self-scheduling administration of pain medications or use of a PCA pump are appropriate choices for the client who is not suffering from confusion or other altered mental states. Positioning and increased activity to reduce complications of immobility and frequent periods of rest is also useful. Client teaching to provide information about the causes of the pain as well as methods for pain relief is important to the elder, affording the potential for even greater control. Finally, consider ethnic or cultural diversity in the expression and meaning of pain, as well as relief alternatives that are specific to the culture of the client. The elderly client may be particularly invested in historical or cultural alternatives. Nonpharmacological methods for pain control that are unacceptable or unbelievable to the client will be of little value. For this reason, client education is essential in successful choice and use of pain control other than or in addition to medication. These choices frequently are more successful in addition to rather than instead of pharmacological pain control.

PAIN MANAGEMENT FOR THE CLIENT WITH ALTERED MENTAL STATUS

Depression and confusion are two changes in mental status that may be seen in the elderly client. Neither of these are normal age-related changes, which are to be expected as part of the aging process. Identifying causes or exacerbating factors and treating the client for depression or confusion should be attempted. However, both confusion and depression may alter the ways in which a client expresses or experiences pain, as well as the efficacy of pain-relief interventions.

Depression may be an organic process or it can be situational. Many clients may experience depression as the result of the diagnosis of an acute or chronic illness, or living with a chronic condition. Depression may also be related to isolation, reduced activity, immobility, or diminished ability for self-care. The client who is depressed appears saddened or presents a flat affect. Changes in eating and sleep patterns occur. Fatigue, loss of energy, and a diminished capacity for enjoyment, peace, or comfort are symptoms as well. The depressed client may not manifest symptoms or complaints about pain as readily. Pain may become quite severe before relief is sought out. For this reason, the client who is depressed should be engaged and assessed repeatedly for pain and the effectiveness of efforts aimed at pain relief. Depression does not cause physical pain, but pain can result in feelings of depression. Chronic pain often has depression as a complicating factor.

Confusion is another mental status change seen in the elderly client. It can be related to a wide variety of client issues. Confusion may have an organic cause, such as Alzheimer's disease or organic brain syndrome. It may result from chronic or acute episodes of hypoxia, sleep deprivation, or be a side effect of medication such as morphine or general anesthesia. Elderly clients are more apt to become confused when removed from a familiar environment or routine. Careful assessment of the client's baseline mental status is important to facilitate removing factors that may cause or exacerbate confusion or forgetfulness. Confusion is commonly assessed initially by orientation to person, place, and time. When disoriented in one or more of these fields, the client may not remember how to seek out relief for pain, what the cause of pain might be, or who has helped with pain-relief interventions.

Assessment criteria for pain in the client with mental status changes differ from those for other clients. Verbal expression of pain or requests for relief may not be evident. The client may not behave as one would expect a client in pain to behave. The depressed client may become even more withdrawn, with a flattened or angry affect. The confused client may exhibit either agitated or withdrawn behavior. Periods of confusion may get longer or the client may appear more confused than his or her baseline assessment. Physical indicators of increased pain may be the only clues. Increases in pulse, respiration, blood pressure; positional changes; guarding; or rigidity of the area of pain, pallor, and diaphoresis are all indicators of pain. Changes in behavior should be considered as indicators of pain. A medication review may indicate potential causes or enhancers of the behavioral changes. Use these cues when deciding to administer pain medication or other interventions, as well as assessing for the effectiveness of interventions provided. Signs and symptoms of pain in the client may be paradoxical and not what you would expect at all. Individualized plans of care for each client include specific assessment criteria and interventions for that particular client.

CUES FOR COMPLIANCE

Interventions for pain relief or a plan of care that include medications as well as non-pharmacological approaches are only useful if the client is compliant with the proposed interventions. Medications that are unavailable, difficult to use, or have intolerable side effects cannot relieve pain when the client opts not to use them. Adjuvant approaches must be believable, available, and easy to use. When designing a pain management program include availability, believability, control, ease of use, and complete and available information.

> Cues for compliance include:
> 1. Available
> 2. Believable
> 3. Easy
> 4. Personal control
> 5. Complete information

When considering availability for the elder client, the health care setting must be considered. In an institutional setting such as hospital or nursing home, the client should understand how to access an intervention through health care personnel. Many elderly clients resist calling the nurse for pain medication, instead waiting until the nurse makes rounds to avoid "bothering" him or her when busy. In this instance, more frequent trips to the bedside or offers for intervention should be a part of the plan of care. Outside of institutional settings, availability includes issues such as affordability of the intervention, where it can be purchased, who will transport it to the client, where it can be safely stored, the client's or family members' ability to administer it safely, and even who can open that child-proof cap!

When designing interventions for pain management, it is important that the client believe that the interventions will help relieve pain. Goals must be realistic. In some instances, complete pain relief is not a realistic option. Communication and understanding of this will help to prevent the client's impression of an intervention as a complete failure. Previous use of medications should be assessed, identifying pain medications that, when used previously, were unsuccessful or problematic. Potential side effects should be planned for from the outset of therapy. Be a cheerleader; help to convince the client that the interventions suggested will be helpful. Continual assessment will identify those interventions that do work. Listen closely to the client's doubts and fears.

Clients who have control over interventions for pain frequently have greater success with pain management. Build control and realistic choices for the client into the plan of care. Self-management of medication, timing, treatment schedules, when and how adjuvant therapies will be used, and who will provide assistance when necessary are all part of the plan. Consider mental status changes when building in appropriate and safe control for the client. Frequent mental status assessment is essential in the elderly client because of increased propensity toward medication-related confusion or sedation. A plan of care is continually evaluated and can be changed frequently as indicated by efficacy.

Interventions that are difficult to accomplish are frequently left unused. The client in pain has diminished energy and resources, and is easily exhausted. This principle is closely related to the discussion of availability above.

Finally, information concerning the interventions planned must be complete and available to the client, significant others, and the whole heath care team. Misunderstanding of incomplete information can be the cause of failure in pain management. Think carefully about documentation techniques and assessment criteria. Verbal, written, and other forms of information are important for the client and significant others, especially as a reference when the nurse is not currently available. Considering details that will increase client compliance will increase the potential for successful pain management.

Case Study Resolved

Mrs. G. no longer verbally complains of pain 5 days after therapy has been instituted. The characteristic rash has not yet resolved, and the nurse notes that her appetite remains diminished and that she is very easily agitated. Mrs. G.'s daughter reports that the client does not engage in conversation and is not interested in watching television. These are unusual for this client. The nurse assesses that Mrs. G. is continuing to have pain, despite the fact that she is not complaining. Medications for pain are changed to an around-the-clock schedule, rather than PRN. Mrs. G. becomes less agitated and less withdrawn. Her appetite improves, and the nurse continues to monitor her bowel status, continuing with the fiber laxative nightly.

BIBLIOGRAPHY

Acute Pain Management Guideline Panel. *Acute Pain Management: Operative or Medical Procedures and Trauma. AHCPR Pub No. 92-0032.* Rockville, Md: Agency for Health Care Policy and Research, Public Health Service, US Department of Health and Human Services; 1992.

American Geriatric Society Panel on Chronic Pain in Older Persons. The management of chronic pain in older persons. *J Am Geriatr Soc.* 1998;46:635-651.

Gagliese L, Melzack R. Chronic pain in elderly people. *Pain.* 1997;70(1):3.

Gagliese L, Katz J, Melzack R. Pain in the elderly. In: Wall PD, Melzack R, eds. *Textbook of Pain.* 4th ed. Edinburgh, UK: Churchill Livingstone; 1999:991-1006.

Galloway S, Turner L. Pain assessment in older adults who are cognitively impaired. *Journal of Gerontological Nursing.* 1999;25(7):34.

Girard N. Care of the geriatric patient. In: Phippen ML, Wells MP, eds. *Patient Care During Operative and Invasive Procedures.* Philadelphia, Pa: WB Saunders; 2000:675-695.

Pasero C, Reed BA, McCaffery M. Pain in the elderly. In: McCaffery M, Pasero C, eds. *Pain: Clinical Manual for Nursing Practice.* 2nd ed. St. Louis, Mo: Mosby; 1999:674-710.

Victor K. Properly assessing pain in the elderly. *RN.* 2001;64(5):45-49.

Young D, Mentes JC, Titler MG. Acute pain management protocol. *Journal of Gerontological Nursing.* 1999;26(5):10.

MULTIPLE-CHOICE QUESTIONS

1. Pain in the elderly population is:
   A. A less frequent problem due to diminished sensation
   B. More common due to increased health care needs
   C. Difficult to manage due to widespread chronic malnutrition
   D. Successfully managed only by gerontology specialists

2. Considerations in choosing a route of administration for medication in the elderly include:
   A. Loss of subcutaneous tissue and muscle mass
   B. Noncompliance
   C. Hearing difficulties
   D. None of the above

3. Manifestations of pain related to vascular changes in the elderly include:
   A. Macular degeneration
   B. Osteoarthritic pain
   C. Intermittent claudication
   D. Pain related to ill-fitting dentures

4. Acute pain in the elderly client:
   A. Is always easily assessed
   B. May be masked by over-the-counter medication use
   C. Is responsive to NSAID therapy
   D. Rarely reflects the severity of illness or trauma

5. Changes in mental status associated with senility, dementia, or Alzheimer's disease may result in inadequate pain management because of:
   A. Masking of manifestations of acute pain
   B. Inability to perceive pain due to central nervous system changes
   C. Inability to vocalize or describe pain
   D. All of the above

6. Narcotic use in the elderly client should be carefully monitored because of which changes in physiology related to aging?
   A. Inability to swallow
   B. Changes in renal function, resulting in faster renal clearance
   C. Changes in liver function, resulting in longer elevated serum drug levels
   D. Restricted mobility, slowing drug metabolism

7. Including analgesic medication in the polypharmacy approach to medication in the elderly includes:

    A. Careful evaluation of all medications currently in use before adding analgesics

    B. Cautioning the elder to take different medications at specified time intervals

    C. Use of multiple pharmacies to fill existing prescriptions

    D. Relying on the elder to coordinate communication among all heath care providers prescribing his or her medications

8. Elderly clients may describe heartburn or symptoms of reflux when using NSAIDs or aspirin therapy. The best intervention to suggest to manage this symptom is:

    A. Take all medications with an 8-ounce glass of milk

    B. Cut tablets in half for easy swallowing

    C. Use enteric coated tablets, if they are available

    D. Restrict use of aspirin or NSAIDs until symptoms disappear

9. Use of heat as a nonpharmacological method of pain management should be monitored carefully because:

    A. An elderly person could easily be electrocuted using a heating pad

    B. An elderly person may be more susceptible to burns because of thin, frail skin and decreased subcutaneous tissue

    C. An elderly client is too confused to remember to use heat

    D. Heat is always the treatment of choice for pain related to vascular insufficiency

10. Which of the following are important to assess with long-term medication intervention for chronic pain?

    A. Mentation

    B. Nutrition

    C. Compliance

    D. All of the above

MULTIPLE-CHOICE ANSWERS

1. B
2. A
3. C
4. B
5. C
6. C
7. A
8. B
9. B
10. D

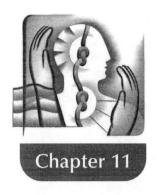

Chapter 11

Treatment of Pain at the End of Life

Case Study 1

S.B. is an 80-year-old female with stage IV breast cancer and metastasis to the bone. She is not a candidate for chemotherapy or radiation and has elected to remain at home without further treatment for her disease. She is being followed by a home hospice agency.

For several months, S.B. has been taking morphine sulfate sustained release (MSSR) 90 mg orally every 12 hours and ibuprofen 200 mg orally every 8 hours to manage low back pain. She occasionally takes morphine sulfate immediate release (MSIR) 30 mg for breakthrough pain. Otherwise, MSSR and ibuprofen control her pain well.

For the past 3 days, S.B. has been extremely weak and fatigued, sleeping most of the day and night, and incontinent of urine. When she is awake she has no desire to eat. The hospice nurse informs the family that the signs and symptoms indicate that her body may be slowing down and that she is likely near death. Given this change in her clinical condition, someone in the home will need to take on the role of managing her medications so that she remains comfortable until death. Medications will also be administered in such a way as to avoid aspiration, which could lead to increased discomfort.

Case Study 2

T.C. is a 74-year-old female with severe chronic obstructive pulmonary disease (COPD), cor pulmonale, osteoporosis, and arthritis. She is dependent on home oxygen and oral steroids. Other medications include diuretics, nonsteroidal anti-inflammatory drugs (NSAIDs), multiple bronchodilators, and respiratory medications. She states that she wants to avoid further hospitalizations for her disease, does not want to be intubated or resuscitated, and that she has a living will and durable power of attorney for health care in place. She is currently being followed by a registered nurse from the transitional care department of a home hospice agency.

For 5 days, T.C. has been on oral antibiotics for acute bronchitis but her overall condition has steadily declined. Today she is lethargic, unable to stand, and having difficulty swallowing her medications. The home care nurse discusses T.C.'s condition with her, her family, and her physician, and they develop a plan of care to keep T.C. at home until she dies.

PAIN IN CLIENTS NEAR DEATH

The literature indicates that unrelieved pain is one of the most common causes of somatic distress in the months, weeks, and days before death.

> The literature indicates that unrelieved pain is one of the most common causes of somatic distress in the months, weeks, and days before death.

Most of what is known about symptoms in individuals near death has been derived from studies on clients with cancer. However, many individuals die from other chronic diseases that are also capable of causing pain and discomfort.

Pain in clients in advanced stages of a life-threatening illness is generally categorized as either nociceptive or neuropathic. Nociceptive pain is transmitted by normal neural activity and represents tissue trauma or inflammation. It can be somatic or visceral in origin, with visceral pain being diffuse, poorly localized, or referred to body surfaces. Neuropathic pain occurs as a result of damage or entrapment of nerves caused by tumor, radiation, or chemotherapy. It characteristically causes burning, the sensation of pins and needles, or electricity-like pain, and is sometimes exacerbated by light touch or temperature changes.

The health care and lay communities are familiar with prognostic estimates for clients with malignant disease. Health care providers also demonstrate an understanding that pain occurs in clients with cancer and that analgesia for pain near death is appropriate. It is questionable, however, how often health care providers utilize prognostic indicators for other chronic, life-threatening disease and how well symptoms such as pain are treated in clients with noncancer diagnoses near death.

The hospice movement has done a great deal to educate people about the process of death and dying, and the need to provide quality end-of-life care.

> It is questionable how often health care providers utilize prognostic indicators for other chronic, life-threatening disease, and how well symptoms such as pain are treated in clients with noncancer diagnoses near death.

Although the majority of clients receiving hospice services have traditionally had a cancer diagnosis, hospice and other palliative care services are not limited to clients with cancer. In 1996, the National Hospice Organization[1] published prognostic guidelines to help identify when individuals with chronic disease other than cancer are in the terminal phase of their disease. Prognostic indicators exist for renal failure, COPD, end-stage cardiac disease, amyotrophic lateral sclerosis, dementia, and acquired immunodeficiency disease (AIDS). Such indicators are not meant to emphasize the negative aspects of chronic disease. Instead, they are meant to assist health care providers in identifying individuals who would likely benefit from services that promote quality of end-of-life care. Despite the availability of these and other measures of prognosis, they are underutilized in guiding treatment at the end of life. The outcome of this is that many individuals near the end of their lives are not provided with quality palliative care, and they are likely to die experiencing pain. Such were the findings of the 1995 Support Study,[2] which looked at factors impacting care for hospitalized adults at the end of life. When death nears, adults with cancer are likely receiving long-acting narcotics to control severe pain. Clients without cancer are less likely to be treated for severe pain and less likely to receive narcotics, particularly long-acting formulas. Because many of these clients are narcotic naïve (ie, have never used narcotic medications), it is likely they will not require the high doses of narcotics that clients with chronic cancer pain require. In fact, clients dying from a cause other than cancer may achieve comfort from pain with non-narcotics and nonpharmacological approaches to pain. What is imperative is that the pain be assessed and treatment be offered, regardless of the etiology. Too often, however, the issue of being near death is not discussed adequately, and assessments for pain and other symptoms of distress are not performed. Perceived risks of medications for pain, such as respiratory depression and lethargy, also act as barriers to treatment, which reinforces the practice of not assessing that which cannot be treated.

> Too often the issue of being near death is not discussed adequately, and assessments for pain and other symptoms of distress are not performed.

Clients with advanced cancer may experience pain throughout the course of their disease. In some situations, treatments such as radiation or chemotherapy can be given to reduce tumor size, resulting in a decrease in pain intensity. Medication, however, is the mainstay of treatment for chronic cancer pain, and the medication is generally given for life to prevent pain from recurring. Adjustments in medication are made if the character of pain changes over time.

As individuals near death, pain may increase, decrease, or remain at the same level of intensity. There are few predictors to identify which clients will experience more or less pain. As death nears, however, clients lose the ability to report and describe their pain because of the lethargy, decreased level of consciousness, or emotional withdrawal accompanying the dying process. The risk that pain will continue or recur and the loss of ability to rely on client reports mandate that medication regimens controlling cancer pain continue with dying clients until death occurs and that alternative methods of assessing pain be implemented.

Just as decreasing or eliminating analgesia in a client with cancer who is near death is not appropriate, it is also not appropriate to decrease or eliminate analgesia in clients near death from a nonmalignant disease. It is not always clear, however, when a client is near death, and signs and symptoms such as a decreased level of consciousness may be attributed to narcotics. In situations where the etiology of a decreased level of consciousness in a client with a life-threatening illness is not clear, the physician may be tempted to decrease or withhold narcotics to assess their role in the change in mental status. The physician should know, however, that clients who have not had significant increases in their narcotics are likely tolerant to the effects of narcotic sedation, and that the narcotics are probably not the cause of their changes in mental status. Caution should be taken in decreasing analgesic dosing in clients near death because of the risk of recurrent pain. Discussion and establishment of the goals of treatment in a client with chronic disease and pain who may be near death should preclude withdrawal of analgesia. Failure to provide adequate treatment to prevent pain puts the client at risk to suffer and die in pain.

The most notable difference in the treatment of pain at the end of life for clients with both malignant and nonmalignant disease is that clients with cancer are more likely to receive narcotics to prevent their pain, often in the long-acting form. Although differences in the pain experience exist, the same guidelines can be used for each client population to facilitate comfort near death.

NONOPIOID ANALGESICS

Nonopioid analgesics include acetaminophen and NSAIDs such as aspirin and ibuprofen. Although often effective for mild to moderate pain of somatic or visceral origin, these drugs have a ceiling effect that limits the amount of the drug that can be administered safely. NSAIDs may also cause adverse effects such as gastrointestinal upset and bleeding. Although clients with rheumatoid arthritis or bone pain often benefit from NSAIDs, histories of gastrointestinal hemorrhage or a low platelet count may make these drugs a poor choice. A thorough assessment of the client's past experiences with pain and analgesics and their side effects is essential to optimal pain management. The experience of pain is somewhat individual, and using analgesics that have been effective for past pain experiences is recommended.

OPIOID (NARCOTIC) ANALGESICS

Pain related to advanced cancer is generally treated with narcotic analgesics. The oral route is preferred because it is relatively safe, noninvasive, easily administered and titrated, and inexpensive. Once pain is controlled, prevention of recurrent pain becomes the goal. Prevention of recurrent pain generally requires administering medication around-the-clock to maintain an adequate level of analgesia. Non-narcotics such as acetaminophen or NSAIDs are the first line of treatment for mild to moderate pain. When pain persists or increases, an opioid such as codeine or hydrocodone is added, often in the form of a combination drug (eg, oxycodone and acetaminophen). Although combination medications are often effective in controlling mild to moderate pain, their use is limited by the content of acetaminophen or NSAID in the medication. For example, 4 grams of acetaminophen is the 24-hour limit for adults. Toxicity could occur with doses exceeding this.

Persistent pain or pain that is moderate to severe in intensity is treated by increasing the opioid potency of drugs. Pure opioid agonists such as morphine, hydromorphone, and oxycodone are the drugs of choice because they do not have a ceiling effect (ie, limited dose requirement). These pure agonists are often given in an extended-release formula to ease administration and prolong control of pain. Medications without a ceiling effect in long-acting formulas include extended-release morphine (eg, MSSR; MS Contin; Oramorph) and controlled or sustained-release oxycodone (eg, Oxycontin SR).

Neuropathic pain may also require adjuvant medications in addition to narcotics. Antidepressants, anticonvulsants, corticosteroids, neuroleptics, and local anesthetics in various doses can enhance analgesic efficacy in specific situations.

CHANGING ROUTES OF ADMINISTRATION NEAR DEATH

A problem with continuing analgesics until death is that clients with a decreased level of consciousness often lose the ability to safely swallow medications, particularly long-acting medications that cannot be chewed or crushed. Alternative routes and dosing schedules to replace analgesics previously taken orally in clients who are no longer able to swallow need to be identified.

Alternative routes and dosing schedules need to be identified to replace analgesics previously taken orally in people who are no longer able to swallow.

Assistance with finding an alternative route generally requires the input of a physician or nurse who is knowledgeable in palliative care. Access to a pharmacist who is able to advise and compound medications for alternative routes is also advantageous.

Short-acting narcotics in liquid form or as crushed tablets may be given sublingually in the buccal mucosa of the cheek or lower lip. The effectiveness of this approach in preventing pain, however, is limited by the amount of the drug that can be given at one time. Clients who have had their pain controlled with only occasional analgesics as opposed to long-acting analgesics may continue to have good control of pain with short-acting analgesics given sublingually. However, clients who have been on high doses of long-acting analgesics likely will require an additional route for administration of medications.

An appropriate alternative route for several long-acting narcotics and non-narcotics is the rectal route. Advantages of this route are that dosing requirements of certain oral medications are the same whether they are administered orally or rectally. Retaining the same dosing requirement eliminates the need to calculate equianalgesic doses and to obtain or purchase new prescriptions. Not only does a switch from oral to rectal administration save family and health care providers time and money, it also facilitates ongoing control of pain by avoiding major changes in the treatment plan.

Although the rectal route is a good alternative for some dying clients, it is not a good alternative for all. Clients with loose stool, constipation, or rectal bleeding may not adequately absorb the analgesia given rectally. Clients with low platelet counts are at risk for bleeding from insertion of medication into the rectum, and clients with lesions of the anus or rectum may experience pain. Rectal administration of analgesics may also pose problems for caregivers who have assumed the responsibility of administering medications near death. Problems cited by family caregivers include aversion to touching the rectum, clients' aversion to having the rectum touched, and difficulty turning the client or inserting the medication into the rectum. It should also be noted that not all oral analgesics can be administered rectally. Assessment for potential problems related to rectal administration of a medication should be made before plans to maintain a client's control of pain are solidified.

Routes of administration of analgesics other than the rectal route are also available to control pain in dying clients with cancer or other pain-related phenomena. The transdermal route is the least invasive alternative route. Use of this route, however, is limited by the number of available analgesics capable of providing relief through transdermal administration, particularly if the analgesia is long acting. Fentanyl is a potent narcotic analgesic that can be used in place of oral analgesia after the appropriate equianalgesic dose is calculated. Transdermal fentanyl, however, should only be used for stable pain, as it is not suitable for rapid dose titration. The decreased blood flow to the skin in a client near death may also impede absorption of this drug. For this reason, clients who are not candidates for rectal administration of long-acting analgesics are usually switched to continuous subcutaneous or intravenous infusions of narcotics to control pain.

Clients are started on intravenous infusions if they have existing intravenous access (eg, central line). If no existing access is available, subcutaneous infusions are generally initiated. The subcutaneous route for continuous administration of narcotics provides blood levels of opiates comparable to those achieved by the intravenous route. Subcutaneous access is also easier to initiate.

Changing a client from the oral route to subcutaneous or intravenous infusion requires calculation of the 24-hour dose of oral analgesia (controlled release and immediate release) and calculation of the equianalgesic dose for the parenteral route. An hourly rate is calculated by dividing the 24-hour total parenteral equianalgesic dose of drug by 24 and dividing that number by 2. Division by 2 is done when first making the change from oral to parenteral to ensure that the dose is not too potent (Table 11-1). Once the parenteral infusion is initiated, the dose can be titrated up as needed to control the pain. Because treatment of pain is often complex, specialists in pain management may be needed to achieve optimal control of pain. Palliative care programs such as hospice often have pain teams composed of experts in pain management who will take referrals or consult by phone with very little notice. These programs also have access to pharmacists and supply companies that can quickly implement a plan of care, even at odd hours, and access to experts in complementary therapies who can engage clients and families in methods to decrease pain. Although physicians and nurses outside of palliative care may be somewhat familiar with complex pain management, clients would benefit more from a comprehensive specialty service that can provide consistent expertise in pain management.

Clients with intractable pain who do not respond to optimal treatment using the therapies described here may require invasive interventions such intraspinal analgesia, nerve blocks, neurosurgery, or surgery to relieve obstruction of a compression that is causing pain.

Case Study 1 Resolved

The route for S.B.'s analgesics needs to be changed from the oral route because she is weak and may have difficulty swallowing the pill and because she should not chew a sustained-release tablet. If acceptable with the client and family, the MSSR can be given rectally, beginning with the same dose as that given orally (90 mg every 12 hours). MSIR must also be made available to administer for breakthrough pain. The liquid form of MSIR, which peaks in 30 minutes, is often preferred over MSIR tablets because it is concentrated and a small amount of fluid can provide substantial analgesia (1 mL = 20 mg; 0.25 mL = 5 mg). Liquid MSIR can be given orally or sublingually in the cheeks. If S.B. were converted from MSIR tablets to MSIR liquid, she would receive 1.5 mL of liquid (20 mg/mL) to equal the 30 mg dose she previously received for breakthrough pain. However, if cost was an issue, the MSIR in tablet form could be given rectally or could be crushed and given sublingually for breakthrough pain. To substitute the oral ibuprofen, a pharmacist can compound the drug in a gel to be given rectally or transdermally in the same dose of 200 mg every 8 hours. Continuing the ibuprofen is particularly important if it is being given for pain related to bone metastasis.

Case Study 2 Resolved

Although T.C. does not have cancer, she has COPD with cor pulmonale, which indicates advanced disease. She has been receiving NSAIDs most likely for pain related to her arthritis and osteoporosis but is no longer able to swallow her medications. A pharmacist can be consulted regarding compounding an NSAID for the rectal or transdermal route (ibuprofen could be used if appropriate). Her respiratory status continues to be managed by inhalation with the appropriate bronchodilators. However, nebulization of these bronchodilators with a mask may be required for optimal absorption of the medication. A small dose of liquid morphine (5 mg = 0.25 mL of a 20 mg/mL concentration) can also be administered to help treat pain or control dyspnea that T.C. is likely to experience. It

Table 11-1

Conversion of Morphine Sulfate from Oral Route to Subcutaneous or Intravenous Route

Step 1. Calculate 24-hour dose of oral narcotic analgesia (controlled release and immediate release)

Add all MS taken in 24 hours:

Example, MS Contin, 90 mg every 12 hours

Immediate release MS, 30 mg (two doses in 24 hours)

   90 mg

   90 mg

+ 60 mg

240 mg of MS (oral dose) in 24 hours

Step 2. Refer to the equianalgesic dosing chart and calculate the equianalgesic dose for the parenteral route.

Morphine:

Oral 30 mg = 10 mg parenteral

$\dfrac{10 \text{ mg}}{30 \text{ mg}} = \dfrac{x}{240 \text{ mg}}$ 30x = 2400

x = 80 mg parenteral dose in 24 hours

Step 3. Divide the 24-hour parenteral dose by 2. (Many consider the parenteral dose on the equianalgesic chart equivalent to an intramuscular dose. Given IV, this would be more potent. Caution should be taken in initiating the change in dose from oral to IV or subcutaneous).

80 ÷ 2 = 40 mg IV or SC in 24 hours

Step 4. Calculate the hourly rate (SC/IV dose) by dividing the 24-hour IV dose by 24.

40 mg ÷ 24 = 1.66 mg each hour or 2 mg each hour

MS = morphine sulfate; IV = intravenous; SC = subcutaneous

should be noted that T.C. is narcotic naïve (ie, she has not been taking narcotics routinely). Thus, she should be started on no more than 5 mg of MSIR orally or sublingually at one time.

CHAPTER SUMMARY

Pain is a common symptom of disease in clients who are near death, regardless of the cause. All health care providers should prioritize the assessment and optimal treatment of pain in clients near death. Treatment generally requires nonopioid or opioid analgesics to prevent the recurrence of known pain and treat escalation or new occurrences. To ensure optimal comfort near death, health care providers must be knowledgeable about alternative routes for analgesia, analgesic dosing, and multiple other issues related to pain near death, or make appropriate and timely referrals to palliative care providers with expertise in the management of pain.

The treatment of pain suggested for the two clients in the case studies is intended to provide an example of a common analgesic plan of care at the end of life. It should be noted, however, that the treatment of pain at the end of life is often complex and optimally involves a more comprehensive assessment, individualized plan of care, and ongoing evaluation of the pain and distress.

REFERENCES

1. National Hospice Organization. *Medical Guidelines for Determining Prognosis in Selected Non-cancer Diseases.* 2nd ed. Arlington, Va: Author; 1996.
2. Support Study Principal Investigators. A controlled trial to improve care for seriously ill hospitalized patients: the study to understand prognoses and preferences for outcomes and risks of treatments (support). *JAMA.* 1995;274(20):1591-1598.

BIBLIOGRAPHY

Coyle N, Layman-Goldstein M. Pain assessment and management in palliative care. In: Matzo ML, Sherman DW, eds. *Palliative Care Nursing: Quality Care at the End of Life.* New York: Springer; 2001:362-486.

Gavrin J, Chapman R. Clinical management of dying patients. *Western Journal of Medicine.* 1995;163:268-277.

Kazanowski M. Symptom management in palliative care. In: Matzo ML, Sherman DW, eds. *Palliative Care Nursing: Quality Care at the End of Life.* New York: Springer; 2001.

Management of Cancer Guideline Panel. *Management of Cancer Pain. Clinical Practice Guidelines. AHCPR Pub No. 94-0592.* Rockville, Md: Agency for Health Care Policy and Research, Public Health Services, US Department of Health and Human Services; 1994.

March PA. Terminal restlessness. *American Journal of Hospice & Palliative Care.* 1998;15(1):51-53.

Paice JA, Fine PG. Pain at the end of life. In: Ferrell BR, Coyle N, eds. *Textbook of Palliative Nursing.* Oxford, UK: Oxford University Press; 2001:76-90.

CASE STUDY QUESTIONS

1. Identify differences and similarities in terms of between the case of S.B. and T.C.
2. Would T.C. require a cancer diagnosis to be admitted on a hospice benefit?
3. Given the information provided, what would you identify as a priority of care for S.B. and T.C.?
4. Given S.B. and T.C.'s difficulty swallowing, the nurse must arrange for what?

MULTIPLE-CHOICE QUESTIONS

1. Which of the following statements about pain near the end of life is accurate:
   A. Pain near death increases only in clients with cancer
   B. Pain is generally not present in the noncancer population
   C. Pain at the end of life is extremely difficult to treat
   D. Pain may increase, decrease, or remain the same as death nears

2. Of the following, which analgesic is limited in terms of the dose that can be administered:
   A. Acetaminophen
   B. Methadone
   C. Morphine sulfate
   D. Oxycontin SR

3. The preferred route for administration of analgesics in a client with mild to moderate pain is:
   A. Intravenous
   B. Oral
   C. Rectal
   D. Transdermal

4. For 3 months John has been receiving Duragesic (fentanyl transdermal system) 50 ucgs for pain related to carcinoma of the lung. John becomes obtunded, difficult to arouse, and is thought to be near death. The nurse should:
   A. Remove the Duragesic patch
   B. Discontinue changing Duragesic patches
   C. Contact the physician
   D. Continue the Duragesic as ordered

5. Which of the following statements about prognostic indicators is accurate:
   A. They are meant to be used only for clients with malignant disease
   B. They assist in identifying individuals who could benefit from end-of-life care
   C. They have no impact on the treatment of pain at the end of life
   D. They have been well-utilized within our health care system

6. Mrs. Jones has been taking MS Contin 60 mg orally every 12 hours for pain related to breast cancer. She has been declining and can no longer swallow. Which of the following interventions is most appropriate:

   A. Start IV morphine at an equianalgesic dose

   B. Start subcutaneous morphine at an equianalgesic dose

   C. Rectal administration of MS Contin

   D. Discontinue MS Contin

CASE STUDY ANSWERS

1. S.B. is a client in hospice, which generally indicates a life expectancy of 6 months or less. S.B. has a malignant disease in advanced stages. T.C. is a client in transitional care. We know nothing about her prognosis, but cor pulmonale is a life-threatening disease.

   S.B's symptoms include lower back pain, which has been well controlled with oral extended-release morphine, ibuprofen, and immediate-release morphine as needed. T.C.'s symptoms are not well defined in the case, but she takes NSAIDS most likely for pain related to her arthritis and osteoporosis.

   S.B.'s symptoms of extreme weakness and fatigue, sleeping incontinence, and anorexia may indicate that she is actively dying. T.C. has acute bronchitis, which is life-threatening to a person with COPD and cor pulmonale. Her lethargy, inability to stand, and difficulty swallowing indicate she is not improving and possibly declining.

   S.B. is a client in hospice, which indicates that she elected to avoid further hospitalization (unless the situation changes) and that someone has likely taken the responsibility of being a primary caregiver. S.B. may or may not have agreed to DNR (do not resuscitate) status, depending on the policy of the particular hospice with which she has contracted. T.C. is not a client in hospice, but she wants to avoid further hospitalizations and she is a DNR.

2. No. Although the majority of clients receiving hospice services have traditionally had a cancer diagnosis, hospice is not limited to clients with cancer. Prognostic indicators also exist for COPD.

3. A priority of care for S.B. and T.C. is comfort (eg, control pain). Both.

4. The nurse must arrange to have appropriate analgesics and other medications for symptoms of distress in the home, which can be given easily to clients who are unable to swallow. S.B. will need to be continued on her MSSR, which can be given rectally. Her MSIR may be given safely in the buccal mucosa, rectally, or transdermally in gel form.

   T.C. may receive ibuprofen in suppository form or in a gel if compounding facilities are available.

MULTIPLE-CHOICE ANSWERS

1. D. Pain may occur in any client near death. Early and ongoing treatment of pain plays a large role in preventing severe pain from occurring at the end of life. The intensity of pre-existing pain may remain the same, may increase, or may decrease as death nears.

2. A. Four grams of acetaminophen is the 24-hour limit for adults. Toxicity could occur with doses exceeding this.

3. B. Oral route is preferred because it is noninvasive, relatively safe, easily titrated, easily administered, and relatively inexpensive. Severe pain that does not respond to oral analgesia may require intravenous analgesics to obtain control. Clients requiring intravenous analgesia are often converted to oral analgesics after control of pain is achieved.

4. D. A decreased level of consciousness is a common manifestation of dying. With a sudden decrease in a client's level of consciousness, health care providers may be tempted to decrease or discontinue narcotics in order to evaluate their possible role in the change in mental status. If there has been no recent increase in narcotic and the client is declining from disease, narcotics are not likely the cause of the mental status change, and they should not be discontinued.

5. B. Prognostic indicators have been underutilized. If they were better utilized, it is believed people near death would more likely receive quality end-of-life care, including quality treatment of pain.

6. C. The rectal route is a good alternative for administration of some long-acting narcotics such as morphine sulfate extended release (eg, MS Contin). The same dose ordered orally can be given rectally, thus eliminating the need to calculate an equianalgesic dose and obtain a different medication. Intravenous infusions may be appropriate if the client has existing intravenous access. However, this would require obtaining a new prescription, the medication for intravenous administration, and appropriate equipment. A less invasive route, such as rectal or transdermal, is generally preferred when clients can no longer swallow. Fentanyl may be appropriate because Mrs. Jones seems to have chronic stable pain. However, it takes 12 to 16 hours for the client to perceive a therapeutic effect and 48 hours to reach a steady state. When initiating Fentanyl in this situation, at least one dose of MS Contin and PRN fast-acting morphine would be given to control the pain until Fentanyl takes effect.

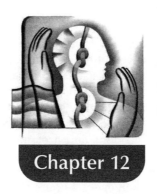

Chapter 12

The Variable Treatment of Pain

Case Study

J.D. is a 34-year-old male who was admitted to the hospital for abdominal pain to rule out peptic ulcer disease. During a diagnostic work-up, a biopsy was taken from tissue in the stomach via upper gastrointestinal endoscopy. The biopsy was found positive for gastric adenocarcinoma. J.D. underwent surgical resection of the stomach under general anesthesia, but the tumor was not completely resected. Postoperatively, J.D. was ordered to receive morphine sulfate 1 mg intravenously (IV) via demand mode of a patient-controlled analgesia (PCA) pump with a lockout interval of 6 minutes and a 4-hour maximum limit of 30 mg.

On the first postoperative night, J.D. rates his abdominal pain as 7 on a scale of 0 to 10 (0 = no pain; 10 = worst pain ever), after receiving 8 mg (ie, eight doses of 1 mg each) of morphine for two consecutive hours. Recognizing that the client's pain is not optimally controlled with near maximum-demand doses, the nurse contacts the surgeon to request an increase in opioid analgesia. The surgeon orders the morphine to be given continuously in addition to demand mode. The dose for the continuous mode is ordered to be 2 mg to 3 mg/hour, and the demand bolus doses are increased to 1.5 mg every 6 minutes. Within an hour, the client reports that his pain has decreased to a level of 4 to 5 using eight boluses without oversedation or respiratory depression. Within 2 hours the client rated his pain 1 to 2 on the continuous hourly rate of 2 mg using one to three demand doses each hour.

On the third postoperative day, the physician decreases the continuous dose of morphine to 1 mg each hour, with a decrease in the bolus to 0.5 mg every 6 minutes as needed (PRN). The client stated that his pain at times is up to 5, usually after activity, but generally responds quickly to demand doses. He continues to receive an hourly continuous infusion and occasional doses (two each shift) of morphine by demand for another 7 days. On the sixth day after surgery, the surgeon discontinues IV morphine, and the client is discharged home. Although the surgeon writes an order for oxycodone 5 mg and acetaminophen 325 mg one to two tablets every 4 hours PRN for pain after the PCA is discontinued, no prescription is written for analgesia after discharge. Discharge orders do, however, include an order for an IV antibiotic to be infused at 8 am daily by a home-health nurse. Arrangements are also made for the client to see a medical oncologist 1 week after discharge for possible treatment of his grade III gastric cancer.

J.D. receives two tablets of oxycodone and acetaminophen (Percocet) in the hospital and is discharged home at 4:30 pm. By 9 pm, the client has severe abdominal pain. J.D.'s wife first calls the surgeon to report the client's severe pain, and the surgeon instructs her to give two tablets of acetaminophen every 4 hours PRN. J.D. receives no relief from the acetaminophen, and his wife contacts the on-call home health nurse.

Because of his diagnosis of advanced gastric cancer, J.D. is admitted to the transitional care/hospice department of the home health agency. Nurses in this department have intensive training in management of pain and embrace the philosophy that pain should be aggressively treated and controlled, particularly with advanced terminal disease. Recognizing that the surgeon did not arrange for analgesia after discharge, the on-call transitional care nurse contacts the medical oncologist who J.D. has an appointment to see next week. Although the oncologist states that he generally does not order medication when he has not yet seen the client, he agrees to order it at this time based on the data provided by the nurse. The nurse instructs the doctor to call the hospice pharmacy, because she knows that the pharmacist there will fill a narcotic with a telephone order from the physician. The oncologist orders morphine sulfate 20 mg/ml, the dose to be 10 to 20 mg orally (PO) PRN every 1 to 2 hours.

UNDERTREATMENT OF PAIN

Lack of effective pain management and wide variability in the management of pain across the health care continuum prompted the federal Agency for Health Care Policy and Research (AHCPR) to study and develop clinical practice guidelines entitled *Acute Pain Management: Operative or Medical Procedures and Trauma*[1] in 1992 and *Management of Cancer Pain: Clinical Practice Guidelines*[2] in 1994. A number of reasons for the inadequate control of pain have been cited in the literature, with the major barriers being 1) misconceptions and attitudes of health care providers toward use of potent narcotics; 2) fear of addiction; and 3) insufficient knowledge of the pharmacology of analgesics.

With the release of the AHCPR guidelines and other concentrated efforts to improve ineffective pain control, there have been improvements in management and control of pain. However, wide variability in knowledge and management continue throughout health care settings. Some of the variability in management of pain seems to be related to the different philosophies of pain management in different practice areas.

> There have been improvements in pain control, but wide variability in knowledge and management continue.

MANAGEMENT OF ACUTE/POSTOPERATIVE PAIN

The *Acute Pain Management: Operative or Medical Procedures and Trauma Clinical Practice Guideline*[1] emphasizes the importance of using an adequate amount of the appropriate analgesia at the appropriate frequency to allow for prolonged analgesia. For the first 48 to 72 hours after most types of major surgery, clients typically require parenteral (ie, intramuscular, subcutaneous, intravenous, or epidural) narcotics to obtain adequate control of pain. Around-the-clock dosing of these opiates are recommended (as opposed to PRN) during the first 24 to 36 hours, with the rationale that pain will be better controlled if analgesia is achieved and the therapeutic level of the drug is maintained.

As the client's pain decreases, the analgesia can be decreased. After 48 hours, many clients may be switched to oral medications that are often less potent. Surgically related postoperative pain should steadily decline 5 to 7 days after surgery, but analgesia with narcotics may be needed for 2 to 3 weeks after surgery for incisional pain. Pain persisting longer than 3 weeks after surgery may indicate a complication of psychological factors that need attention.

Ineffective control of postoperative pain commonly occurs when health care providers switch a client from parenteral narcotics to oral narcotics, which generally are not as potent. Ineffective control of pain also occurs when oral opioids are ordered at a frequency that does not relate to their duration of action (eg, medication with analgesic duration of 3 hours is ordered every 4 hours PRN).

> Ineffective control of postoperative pain commonly occurs when health care providers switch a client from parenteral narcotics to oral narcotics, which are generally not as potent.

Case Study Revisited

In the case of J.D., his postoperative pain was somewhat responsive to morphine but not adequately controlled with the dose given via the demand mode of a PCA pump. The increase in the dose of the PRN medication (from 1 mg to 1.5 mg) and the increase in the frequency accomplished by the continuous mode led to much better pain control within 2 hours of initiating the change. When the continuous dose of morphine was decreased from 2 mg to 1 mg an hour on the third postoperative day, the client continued to have good control of pain. Although at times he rated his pain a 5, it generally occurred with activity (that often increases over time), and the pain continued to be quickly relieved with demand doses of morphine. Thus, J.D.'s pain seemed to be managed adequately until the sixth postoperative day when the continuous and demand doses were abruptly discontinued and replaced with an oral narcotic of much less potency and limited to two doses, with no narcotic analgesia available after the client was discharged.

To prepare postoperative clients for discharge, parenteral medications are commonly switched to oral medications because the route is more convenient for self-management after discharge. However, practitioners need to consider how potencies of parenteral medications relate to potencies of oral medications. AHCPR guidelines recommend the use of an equianalgesic chart to determine how a certain amount of drug given via a certain route compares in potency to the same drug given by another route or a different drug (see Chapter 3).

In postoperative clients, it is generally expected that pain will decrease and that analgesia will decrease as the client recovers. This may also be the expectation for other clients in the acute care setting who have not undergone surgery. This should not, however, be the expected outcome for every client.

A client who has been receiving only an occasional dose of IV or intramuscular (IM) morphine may tolerate a change to an oral narcotic (thus, a decrease in potency of the dose). A client requiring IM or IV doses of morphine every 3 hours will not likely tolerate a change to oral narcotics unless the change is equianalgesic. For example, 10 mg of morphine sulfate given IM is equivalent to 30 mg of oral morphine. Therefore, if a client required eight doses of morphine at 10 mg each over a 24-hour period of time (ie, every 3 hours), any equivalent less than 30 mg of oral morphine every 3 hours would be a decrease in analgesia.

Practitioners in acute care do not routinely order an equianalgesic dose of narcotics when switching routes. More typically, an oral narcotic such as 5 to 10 mg of oxycodone (with or without acetaminophen) is ordered. Many postoperative clients tolerate the change in dose well, particularly when the narcotic is combined with a non-narcotic analgesic such as acetaminophen (eg, Percocet or Tylox). Clients with severe pain will not, however, tolerate the change.

When practitioners anticipate that a client being switched from parenteral narcotics to oral narcotics may have less than adequate pain relief, parenteral narcotics should be ordered as a "back-up." Clients who require frequent dosing with parenteral analgesics prior to switching to an oral narcotic may have better pain control if they are given oral narcotics around the clock (as opposed to PRN).

Case Study Revisited

From the third to the sixth postoperative day, J.D. received a continuous dose of 1 mg of intravenous morphine hourly, with demand doses of 0.5 mg approximately twice each shift (six times in 24 hours). The total amount of morphine he received each of these days was 27 mg intravenously. A dose of 27 mg intravenous morphine is equivalent to three times that amount (81 mg) orally. When the route of J.D.'s morphine was changed, he could have received up to 60 mg oxycodone (equivalent to 20 mg morphine and 3750 mg acetaminophen PRN) in 24 hours. He was in the hospital, however, only long enough to receive one dose (10 mg oxycodone/625 mg acetaminophen) before being discharged home. The initial change in route and decrease in analgesia may have been appropriate if J.D. had remained hospitalized with ready access to more potent opioids for back-up. However, a dramatic decrease in opioid without an available narcotic for intermittent pain in a client with an unresectable gastric tumor is inappropriate.

Development of a Discharge Pain Management Program

As described, J.D. developed severe abdominal pain on the first night after discharge from the hospital. When the transitional care/hospice nurse is called about his pain, she questions why it was that J.D.'s plan of discharge did not include at least a mild narcotic. The nurse notes that J.D. has a diagnosis of advanced gastric cancer and that he has been referred to the transitional care department of home care, which commonly follows clients with advanced malignant disease. The nurse also notes that 24 hours prior to discharge, the client required parenteral narcotics to control his pain but now has no narcotics ordered. Additionally, she notes that J.D. has a documented history of drug abuse. The transitional care nurse knows that J.D.'s pain is severe, and it will require a strong narcotic for relief. The documented history of drug abuse cues her to consider that J.D. may require a higher dose of narcotics to relieve his pain because of past intolerance to opiates.

One can only hypothesize why J.D. was sent home with such an inadequate plan for pain management. It is likely that the discharge plan of care was based on the rationale (and acute care mindset) that the pain of recovering postoperative clients is expected to decrease. However, such a mindset does not take into account the fact that an unresected tumor could contribute to his pain. A thorough assessment of the client's pain prior to discharge might have yielded more comprehensive information, and it may have cued the physician or nurse that J.D.'s pain was of malignant origin. Pain of malignant origin is not likely to decrease, and it needs to be treated after discharge. If the physician had any question about the etiology of the pain, the oncologist could have been consulted prior to discharge or a narcotic analgesic could have been prescribed.

Another factor that might have played a role in J.D.'s discharge plan is his history of drug abuse. Unlike the hospice nurse who saw the client's history as a reason to provide adequate (and possibly high) doses of analgesia, practitioners in acute care often view the history of drug abuse as a reason to withhold narcotics. In some states, physicians must report narcotic prescriptions to known drug abusers to the federal authorities. Physicians are reluctant to order narcotics for clients with this history because of their obligation to report and because of the perception that providing narcotics to known abusers will promote addiction.

It is possible that the surgeon and the nurse discharging the client home did not believe the client would have severe pain after discharge. The surgeon and nurse may also have assumed that the oncologist and transitional care nurse would monitor and manage the pain. Indeed, the transitional care nurse's involvement did lead to a resolution. It is, however, likely that the nurse and physician lacked knowledge of the needs and barriers to pain management that clients with pain face in the home.

Clients are often physically and emotionally isolated from the health care community. Clients and families often avoid contacting health care providers because of their discomfort talking to providers and their beliefs that they will be perceived as complainers. Even clients and families who are able to communicate with health care providers face barriers to management of pain. Not all pharmacies accept a telephone order for opiates, and those that will accept one reserve the right to refuse such an order. If the pharmacy does not accept a telephone order, families and clients often need to: 1) wait until a physician writes a prescription for analgesia; 2) to arrange pick-up of the prescription from the physician; and 3) bring the prescription to a pharmacy that has the medication in stock. Another barrier to the treatment of pain for clients in the home is the third-party payment system for prescription drugs. Many insurance providers require that medications be purchased only in those pharmacies with which they have contracted. A pharmacy that is willing to accept a telephone order may not accept the clients' medication card, may not be convenient for the family, or may have limited hours of operation.

All of these barriers can delay the treatment of pain, which when left untreated often escalates to a level at which it is difficult to control. The negative impact of these barriers on the treatment of pain cannot be overstated, and every effort should be taken to avoid putting a client in such a situation. Health care providers in both acute care and outpatient or chronic care settings should do everything they can to ensure that a client at risk for having pain has a workable plan in place, which at the very least includes access to effective analgesia. In this age of managed care, where so many clients are sick in their homes and where visits to emergency departments are discouraged (and not approved), both nurses and physicians must look upstream, planning for what may occur when the client is home. Potential problems such as pain also need to be recognized and treated as priorities.

CHAPTER SUMMARY

Within our health care system there is wide variability in the management of pain, often related to areas of practice and different philosophies of care. Multiple barriers to effective treatment abound, but those who prioritize client comfort are able to overcome the barriers to achieve the goal. Hospice care is considered the leader in pain management practice, and health practitioners who are affiliated with hospice and palliative care have embraced the philosophy that pain should be treated adequately in all clients with terminal disease, regardless of the obstacles.

Client problems and needs are difficult to predict, but practitioners must strive to plan as comprehensively as possible for all clients being discharged from their service. The potential for a client having pain must be given high priority, even with concerns such as drug abuse. An interdisciplinary team should be consulted if concerns such as drug abuse block effective pain management.

> The potential for a client having pain must be given high priority, regardless of concerns such as drug abuse.

Case Study Resolved

J.D. did not have ready access to effective analgesia after discharge from acute care. However, his physician arranged for follow-up with an oncologist and home hospice nurse who ultimately facilitated the management of his pain.

The resolution of J.D.'s pain primarily came about because the home health nurse from transitional care/hospice prioritized the need to treat the client's pain promptly and did not allow any barriers to block this intervention. It was the nurse who recognized that the J.D.'s pain was severe and immediately implemented a plan of care to obtain the appropriate medication promptly, despite the fact that it was midnight. The nurse knew what medication would likely relieve the client's pain safely yet promptly, knew what medications could be safely given in the home, and knew a pharmacist who could accept an emergency phone order for analgesia and fill the order immediately. The nurse then phoned the oncologist, who ordered the appropriate analgesia promptly and arranged for the medication to be picked up. The nurse then went to the client's home to assist him and his family with administration of the medication, and instruct them on additional analgesia orders until the pain could be reassessed and the physician could be contacted in the morning.

The philosophy of hospice care is to prioritize clients' comfort, and because poor pain and symptom management is known to be a problem, the agency where this hospice nurse was employed had a plan in place to address situations such as J.D.'s. But the key to success was not only in the plan—the key to J.D.'s relief of pain was also a result of the nurse's perception of the pain as unacceptable and her commitment to facilitating prompt pain relief and control. The nurse needed to identify a physician who would order appropriate medication. The nurse also recognized the need to arrange for payment and delivery of the medication, because J.D.'s family did not have the resources for either.

> The key to J.D.'s relief of pain was also a result of the nurse's perception of the pain as unacceptable and her commitment to facilitating prompt relief and control.

J.D.'s pain responded well to liquid oral morphine sulfate that the nurse administered in increments of 5 to 10 mg every 10 minutes, for a total of two doses (20 mg). The physician ordered morphine sulfate 20 mg/1 mL by mouth every 1 to 2 hours PRN for pain. Although the nurse monitored the client's respiratory rate and level of sedation, she knew that the client recently had tolerated continuous and demand doses of intravenous morphine, which is at least three times as potent as oral morphine. As expected, J.D. tolerated 20 mg of oral morphine given over 15 minutes. The hospice nurse also knew that because the client's pain was so severe, J.D. would likely require a high dose of analgesia to get the pain under control. J.D. stated his pain decreased from a level of 10+ to a level of 8 within 10 minutes after receiving the initial dose of 10 mg oral morphine. Within 2 hours, after receiving a total of 40 mg of oral morphine, the client rated his pain as 1 to 2 and stated he was comfortable.

Recognizing that the client's pain would likely increase without long-acting or continuous morphine, the nurse instructed the client to begin taking 5 to 10 mg of morphine each hour and to take up to 20 mg every hour if needed. The nurse arranged for the day nurse to visit the client at 8 am to reassess his pain, evaluate the medication treatment plan, and contact the physician about implementing a long-acting analgesic if the pain was expected to continue.

REFERENCES

1. Acute Pain Management Guideline Panel. *Acute Pain Management: Operative or Medical Procedures and Trauma Clinical Practice Guideline.* AHCPR Pub No. 92-0032. Rockville, Md: Agency for Health Care Policy and Research, Public Health Service, US Department of Health and Human Services; 1992.
2. Management of Cancer Pain Guideline Panel. *Management of Cancer Pain: Clinical Practice Guidelines.* AHCPR Pub No. 94-0592. Rockville, Md: Agency for Health Care Policy and Research, Public Health Service, US Department of Health and Human Services; 1994.

BIBLIOGRAPHY

American Pain Society. *Principles of Analgesic Use in the Treatment of Acute Pain and Cancer Pain.* 4th ed. Glenview, Ill: American Pain Society; 1999.

Ferrell B, McCaffery M, Rhiner, M. Pain and addiction: an urgent need for change in nursing education. *J Pain Symptom Manage.* 1992;7:48-55.

McCaffery M, Ferrell BR. Nurses' knowledge of pain assessment and management: how much progress have we made? *J Pain Symptom Manage.* 1997;14:175-188.

CASE STUDY QUESTIONS

1. What should have been the goal for J.D.'s pain on the first postoperative night?
2. What should have been the goal for J.D. after discharge?
3. How much pain would be expected for J.D. on his day of discharge?
4. J.D., with a diagnosis of gastric cancer and pain, is discharged home without narcotic analgesia. Recurrence of the pain will negatively affect his quality of life and functional status. Name two other problems that could occur after discharge with regard to his pain.

MULTIPLE-CHOICE QUESTIONS

1. Lack of effective pain control in this country is attributed to all of the following *except*:
    A. Fear of addiction
    B. Insufficient knowledge of analgesic pharmacology
    C. Misconceptions about potent narcotics
    D. The Agency for Health Care Policy and Research

2. According to AHPCR clinical practice guidelines for acute pain, for the first 24 to 36 hours postoperatively, clients should receive analgesics:
    A. Around the clock
    B. Orally
    C. PRN (as needed)
    D. Intravenously

3. Which of the following would be an equianalgesic dose for 10 mg of intramuscular morphine:
    A. Morphine sulfate 10 mg tablet
    B. Morphine sulfate 30 mg tablet
    C. Oxycodone 5 mg tablet
    D. Oxycodone 10 mg tablet

4. When a postoperative client's analgesics are changed from the parenteral to the oral route, the dose is usually:
    A. Decreased
    B. Increased
    C. Kept the same
    D. Determined by the patient's needs

5. M.J. is 5 days post total hip replacement. Her pain is well-controlled with MS 10 mg IM every 4 hours. Her physician elects to discontinue the parenteral morphine. Which of the following is the best plan of care for M.J.?

   A. A non-narcotic oral analgesic PRN (as needed)

   B. Around-the-clock narcotic oral analgesia, a scheduled non-narcotic oral analgesic, and parenteral narcotics as back-up

   C. Narcotic oral analgesia PRN

   D. Scheduled oral steroids

CASE STUDY ANSWERS

1. Relief of pain, with pain rating of 0 to 2 (on a 0 to 10 scale with 0 being no pain and 10 being most severe pain possible) or at a level with which the client is satisfied without respiratory depression or oversedation.

2. Pain rated 0 to 2 with optimal function.

3. This may be difficult to determine, but the surgeon should be able to give some idea of how much tumor remained postoperatively and how much pain could be attributed to that versus incisional pain. Even without this information, the nurse preparing the client for discharge needs to perform a thorough assessment of J.D.'s pain and calculate how much opioid he required the day prior to discharge in an effort to determine the minimum amount he would require 1 day later.

4. Without ready access to analgesics to treat pain in early stages, J.D. will not be able to treat his pain when it initially occurs. Without prompt treatment, his pain may escalate to a point where it is very difficult to control, and he may need to go to the ER, with possible re-admission to the hospital.

MULTIPLE-CHOICE ANSWERS

1. D. The AHCPR developed clinical practice guidelines for acute pain and cancer pain. These guidelines have led to improvements in pain control.

2. A. Pain will be better controlled if a therapeutic level of analgesia is maintained.

3. B. Analgesics given parenterally are generally more potent than analgesics given orally. Oxycodone 30 mg would be equivalent to 10 mg morphine IM.

4. A. Practitioners in acute care do not routinely order an equianalgesic dose of narcotics in postoperative clients when switching from parenteral to oral routes.

5. B. A client requiring parenteral narcotics every 4 hours will not likely tolerate a change to oral analgesics. Addition of a non-narcotic will likely help, but the oral narcotics should also be given around the clock with parenteral narcotics used as back-up.

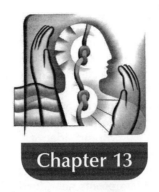

Strategies to Assist Family Caregivers Treating Pain and Suffering at the End of Life

Case Study

M.B. is a 40-year-old woman with advanced lung cancer whose tumor has not responded to recent chemotherapy and whose overall condition is declining. When told of her condition, she requests to go home to die. A referral to home hospice is made.

On the first home visit, the nurse finds M.B. to be extremely lethargic with cool, clammy skin. She is awake enough to answer simple questions and admits to pain and nausea. She is moaning at rest, and she grimaces with movement. At the start of the visit, M.B.'s mother is the only person in the house. She tells the nurse that she gave Percocet to her daughter for pain, and she is able to identify all of her medications, including the new symptom relief kit ordered by the doctor. M.B.'s husband enters the room but stands in the back, away from the client. He has tears in his eyes and his overall appearance is of sadness and shock.

The nurse tells M.B., her mother, and her husband that she would like to see her more comfortable, and she offers to administer an antiemetic suppository and liquid morphine for pain. The nurse administers a 25 mg suppository of prochlorperazine and 0.5 ml (10 mg) of liquid morphine (sublingually). Recognizing that M.B. will require symptom management after she leaves, the hospice nurse offers to develop a medication plan to manage M.B.'s pain and nausea and to plan for other symptoms that could occur. M.B.'s mother collaborates in the plan but states that she will only be available during the day. M.B.'s husband admits he'll be in the home when his mother-in-law leaves, listens to the nurse's recommendations for medication, but says, "I don't think I can do this."

FAMILY CAREGIVERS

With the shift in health care delivery from the hospital to the home and the availability of home hospice services, more clients are being cared for in the home near the end of life. Although home care nurses may be referred to coordinate, monitor, evaluate, and revise plans of care, the time nurses spend in the home is limited by third-party payment systems. Family and friends in the home are required to assume the responsibility for providing the majority of direct client care. Direct client care includes management that requires caregivers to recognize symptoms, identify the appropriate treatment, and administer the medication by oral, sublingual, transdermal, or rectal route. Any one component of this process can be unfamiliar and anxiety-provoking to a lay person, particularly given the changing nature of symptoms near death.

> When a client chooses to die at home, family and friends are required to assume the responsibility for providing the majority of direct client care.

Families vary in how they organize and provide caregiving. However, most select one person who assumes the role.[1] Because the role involves a 24-hour-a-day commitment, others may need to assist. The majority of primary caregivers in the home have traditionally been women.[2] The trend, however, is that males are increasingly taking on the caregiver role.

Skills to make decisions about management of symptoms are not inherent in lay caregivers. Although instructions on symptom management can be taught, lay caregivers lack the clinical judgment that health care professionals have acquired through education and experience to assess and treat symptoms of distress. Lay caregivers may not recognize symptoms of distress. If able to identify symptoms, they may be reluctant to give medication to treat symptoms for a variety of reasons. At the same time that they are monitoring clients and making decisions on treatment of symptoms, family caregivers are also dealing with the psychosocial and emotional impact related to the loss of the client's health and independence, and anticipating the loss they will feel after the client's death. Symptom management in a stable situation when clients are near death can be difficult enough, but the sudden onset of new symptoms and intensification of old symptoms can render the task even more difficult; and crisis may occur.

Studies have shown that caregivers have difficulty making decisions about the management of pain in clients in the home both before the terminal phase[3] and near the client's death.[4]

Difficulties arise when clients can no longer verbally report their symptoms or collaborate on decisions to treat; when caregivers perceive that the client would prefer to defer taking treatment for a symptom; and when family members object to treatment of a symptom, administration of a certain medication such as morphine, or the use of a particular route such as rectally. Another barrier to caregiver treatment of symptoms is fear of overdosing or harming the client.

Whereas some factors act as barriers to treatment of symptoms near death, other factors can facilitate caregiver treatment. Factors that facilitate treatment work by prompting the caregivers to administer a medication. Facilitating factors include receiving information on management of symptoms from a home hospice provider, instruction regarding which symptoms are more likely to occur (related to the disease and to past client experiences), ongoing interaction with the nurse and reliance on the hospice nurse's judgment, the ability of the client to verify presence of a symptom, past experience observing a specific symptom, recognition of client behavior associated with a symptom (eg, reaching for emesis basin when nauseated), and perception that the symptom indicates suffering.

It is important to note that influences on caregiver decisions to treat symptoms near death will vary in their effect among caregivers and vary as situations and circumstances change. It is not the simple presence or absence of a factor that will predict caregiver decisions to treat. It is the effect that a factor has on a caregiver at a certain point in time and in a certain place. Though knowledge of potential influences on management of symptoms is helpful in identifying potential caregiver difficulties and strengths, this knowledge is limited by its relation to the particular context of the situation and by its interaction with other influencing factors.

PAIN AND SYMPTOMS OF DISTRESS AT THE END OF LIFE

Most of what is known about the occurrence and treatment of symptoms near death has come from studies of clients with terminal cancer. Research has identified up to 44 symptoms known to occur near death, with pain, dyspnea, delirium, nausea, and vomiting considered the most distressing for clients to endure. Although the distinction for pain is generally made, symptoms such as dyspnea and delirium can cause suffering that is equal to or greater than some types of pain. It is therefore important that these other symptoms be included in discussions related to pain at the end of life.

> Research has identified up to 44 symptoms known to occur near death, with pain, dyspnea, delirium, nausea, and vomiting considered the most distressing for clients to endure.

Like pain near death that can intensify, decrease, or remain the same, so can dyspnea, delirium, nausea, and vomiting. Often, these symptoms need to be treated aggressively to prevent their escalation. Effective management and control of symptoms near death can be achieved more than 90% of the time when the client has access to experts in palliative care. Even with optimal care, a small percentage of clients will likely have intractable symptoms that may require sedation until death.

> Health care providers may initiate discussions with clients and family that empathize the value of having medications available in the home should symptoms of distress occur.

Family caregivers of clients known to be in advanced stages of a terminal illness should have plans in place to treat symptoms of distress when a client's condition begins to decline. It is very difficult to predict when clients with terminal illness will actually die, and discussions about dying are often avoided by health care providers so as not to upset clients and family. A plan for ensuring that a small amount of medication is readily available should symptoms occur suddenly can prevent undue pain and suffering. Having medication accessible is especially important for clients who wish to remain in their homes until death. To address this need, some hospices have developed what they call symptom relief kits that are made up of a variety of medications commonly prescribed for pain, dyspnea, agitation, nausea, and vomiting. The medications in these kits are generally in a form that can be administered by lay caregivers to clients who are unable to swallow. For example, morphine is usually supplied as a liquid solution that can be given in small amounts sublingually in the cheeks or in front of the lower gum line. Levsin for excessive oral secretions is provided

Some hospices have developed what they call symptom relief kits that are made up of a variety of medications commonly prescribed for pain, dyspnea, agitation, nausea, and vomiting.

as a very small tablet, which can be crushed and with a drop of water, placed under the tongue or in the cheeks. Most of the other medications in the kit are in a suppository form, which lay caregivers often can administer without difficulty. Medications that require RN administration may also be added to the kit, because most hospice agencies have an RN on call who could administer the medication if needed. Only small amounts of medications are placed in the kit in an effort to minimize costs while allowing treatment for a variety of symptoms. Medications in the kit generally provide 12 to 16 hours of symptom management to allow relief until additional medications can be ordered and obtained. Development of such kits requires collaboration among pharmacists, nurses, and physicians to determine what medications should be included and how kits should be ordered and used in practice.

Development of symptom relief kits requires collaboration among pharmacists, nurses, and physicians to determine which medications should be included and how kits should be ordered and used in practice.

Table 13-1 summarizes the contents of one home hospice's symptom relief kit. Use of this kit has facilitated prompt and effective relief of symptoms for many clients, while avoiding uncomfortable and costly emergency room visits or hospitalizations. Nurses admitting clients to home hospice or palliative care programs should ideally arrange to have such kits prescribed and delivered to homes prior to the onset or intensification of a distressful symptom such as pain.

Though clients with terminal cancer make up the majority of hospice referrals, clients with terminal conditions such as end-stage heart disease, chronic obstructive pulmonary disease, Alzheimer's disease, or amyotrophic lateral sclerosis are also hospice-appropriate. Clients with each of these illnesses have been shown to benefit from ready access to symptom relief kits.

INSTRUCTING FAMILY CAREGIVERS ON SYMPTOM MANAGEMENT

Before instructing family members on how to manage a client's pain or symptoms of distress near death, the nurse needs to assess the family's understanding of the situation and their feelings about the client experiencing pain. The nurse then instructs caregivers to ask the client if he or she is having pain and/or dyspnea at least every few hours and/or assess for objective signs of pain or distress (ie, grimacing, moaning, restlessness, confusion). Caregivers should not rely on clients to report pain or dyspnea on their own. Ideally, the caregiver should measure the intensity of the pain or dyspnea using a method that both the client and caregiver can easily understand and implement. The simplest method involves rating the symptom from 0 to 10, with 0 indicating no pain or dyspnea and 10 indicating the worst pain or dyspnea possible. Clients may not be able, however, to use numeric ratings to conceptualize or communicate intensity of symptoms, particularly as death nears. In these situations, caregivers need not be concerned with rating the pain but should instead focus on watching the client for any symptom of distress and medicating the client based on the presence of the distress. Times, types, and amounts of

Table 13-1

Symptom Relief Kit

Symptom	Medication	Dosage
For unrelieved pain	Morphine sulfate solution 20 mg/ml	1-2 ml (PO/SL) if taking long-acting opioids q 2-3 hrs PRN 0.25-0.5 ml (PO/SL) if opioid naive q 2 hrs PRN
For unrelieved dyspnea	Morphine sulfate solution 20 mg/ml	0.25-0.5 ml (PO/SL) q 2 hrs PRN for dyspnea or shortness of breath
For nausea or vomiting	Prochlorperazine (compazine)	25 mg suppository 1 pr q 8 hrs PRN
For restlessness, nausea, or vomiting	ABH (Ativan 1 mg, Benadryl 12.5 mg, Haldol 1 mg)	1 suppository q 8 hrs PRN
For agitation and restlessness: • Determine if client is in pain; treat accordingly • Determine if client is constipated or having urinary retention; take appropriate action • If agitation persists and safety of client or caregiver is at risk, administer	Pentobarbital (hyoscyamine)	60 mg suppository 1 q 4-6 hrs PRN
For loud, wet respirations or excessive secretions	Levsin 0.125 mg	1-2 tablets (PO/SL) q 4-6 hrs PRN
For unrelieved respiratory fluid accumulation or unrelieved dyspnea	Furosemide	40-80 mg IV, SC, or IM
For fever	Acetaminophen 650 mg	1 suppository q 4 hrs PRN

PO = by mouth; SL = sublingual; IV = intravenous; SC = subcutaneous; IM = intramuscular
Reprinted with permission from VNA Hospice, Optima Health Visiting Nurse Services, Manchester, NH.

medications administered should be written down in a diary or central log to which other family members and professional caregivers have ready access. This diary is used to evaluate the effectiveness of symptom management over time and to adjust medication schedules when necessary.

Family caregivers have described multiple uncertainties when managing medications for a client in the home, and it is known that they do not administer as-needed medications as frequently as they could be used. To facilitate medication management of a client's pain, a plan to manage pain should minimize the frequency with which caregivers are faced with decision making and optimize the control of pain and other symptoms of distress. Long-acting opioids often accomplish the goal of minimizing dosing and controlling pain. However, long-acting opioids are not initiated until clients require and demonstrate tolerance to a certain amount of narcotic. Initially, opioids are initiated in short-acting doses, with an increase in frequency when needed. Symptoms such as dyspnea, nausea, vomiting, and delirium are also initially treated with short-acting doses of medications. Although these medications are most often prescribed to be used every few hours as needed, it is prudent that the nurse consider routine scheduling of appropriate as-needed medications to facilitate better symptom control. For example, clients who begin to have dyspnea may be scheduled to receive immediate-release morphine sulfate 5 mg SL every 2 hours around the clock, as opposed to every 2 hours PRN.

It is known that family caregivers committed to a client's comfort until death can effectively manage medications for a dying person's pain in the home. Family caregivers, however, report that they need the information and ongoing clinical support that an expert in end-of-life care (eg, hospice nurse) provides to accomplish this. Not only do family caregivers rely on the assistance a hospice nurse when they initially become involved in the management of pain in the home, caregivers have also stated that they rely on the ongoing assessments and reinforcement of instructions related to administering medications that the nurse provides on visits to the home throughout the dying process. The interaction with the hospice nurse on each visit provides caregivers with the reassurance that they are making accurate assessments and giving appropriate care. It is important that family believe they have provided safe, effective care to their loved ones not only during the period of symptom management but also after the client's death.

The experience of managing a person's pain near death is a process that continues to be experienced even after the client's death. Despite having administered safe amounts of analgesic to promote comfort, family caregivers have reported that they sometimes experience guilt when they reflect on their medication management of symptoms, even after the client's death. This experience of guilt is likely to occur when caregivers have been in the role of managing medications for a short period of time and/or when the client died after the caregiver administered morphine.

Strategies to help identify barriers or facilitating factors for treatment of symptoms include assessing caregivers for fears, conflicts, their perception of symptoms related to suffering, and past client perceptions of medications. The hospice nurse should instruct caregivers regarding which symptoms of distress are most likely to occur based on the client's diagnosis and past symptoms. The hospice nurse should also visit clients experiencing changes in symptoms and/or changes in treatment daily and visit clients with stable symptoms at least every 2 days to assess, review medication management plans, and verify medication plans with caregivers to reassure them that they are managing symptoms well. Nurses should assess caregiver needs by phone at least daily when clients are known to be near death, and caregivers should have 24-hour access to a hospice provider who is familiar with the client's situation.

CHAPTER SUMMARY

Individuals near death are at risk for symptoms of distress, the most frequently cited being pain, dyspnea, restlessness, and labored breathing. Efforts to assess and promptly treat any of these symptoms are essential if suffering near death is to be prevented. Family caregivers are expected to monitor clients in the home and treat symptoms of distress near death. Though they are not professional health providers, with the appropriate information and ongoing clinical support from experts in palliative care, family caregivers are able to effectively manage symptoms near death.

Case Study Resolved

During her initial visit to M.B.'s home, the nurse assessed that her mother was the primary caregiver and manager of medications, but that she was only in this role during the day. She assessed that M.B. was experiencing pain and nausea, and that she had a short episode of dyspnea on exertion. The nurse verified that the family was aware that M.B. was near death and discussed the goal of comfort. After reviewing and verifying that M.B.'s mother and her husband were able to identify the symptom relief kit and other medications, the nurse demonstrated which medications to give for the nausea and for pain, and how to give each. She administered a 25 mg prochlorperazine suppository from the symptom relief kit, which was prescribed PRN for nausea or vomiting. Although M.B. had been taking Percocet for pain, her pain continued. The nurse suggested that M.B. try the liquid morphine sulfate in the symptom relief kit. Morphine is more potent, quicker acting, easier to swallow, and easier to administer than a pill. The nurse administered the liquid morphine sublingually in the client's cheek (oral mucosa). Within 15 minutes, M.B.'s pain and nausea were greatly relieved.

Recognizing that the nausea and pain would likely recur if medications were not routinely administered, the nurse developed a medication plan in writing to include administration of a prochlorperazine suppository (antiemetic) at least every 8 hours, and analgesia (liquid morphine sulfate 10 mg) at least every 3 hours. Based on M.B.'s diagnosis of lung cancer and her dyspnea with activity, the nurse knew that she was a risk for having dyspnea occur as death neared. To further assess the risk, the nurse auscultated M.B.'s lungs and assessed for edema. Because her lungs were clear with no edema and because M.B. denied shortness of breath at rest, the nurse did not include specific medication for dyspnea in the scheduled medication plan.

Noting that M.B.'s mother would be leaving and her husband would likely assume the caregiver role, the nurse turned her attention to him. She recognized that he was afraid and anxious based on his statements, "I don't think I can do this," and "I cannot give a suppository." Recognizing that the husband also wanted to fulfill his wife's request to die at home, the nurse asked M.B.'s mother if there was any family member or friend that could stop by the house briefly at 10 pm and administer another suppository. M.B.'s sister was contacted and agreed to do this. M.B.'s husband said that he could give the morphine solution, and her mother stated she would give the next scheduled antiemetic suppository when she returned in the morning.

To minimize M.B.'s pain and dyspnea with activity, the nurse offered to insert a Foley catheter, to which the client agreed. A home health aid was assigned to visit the client early each morning, and she agreed to assume most of the catheter care. The nurse eliminated medications that were no longer necessary for symptom management, repeated instructions regarding the scheduled medications for nausea and pain, and instructed the family that extra doses of morphine solution could be given hourly if needed for pain or shortness of breath. The husband and mother were instructed to call hospice if pain, nausea, or dyspnea was not relieved by the medications, and/or if the client became agitated, restless, or exhibited other symptoms of distress. The nurse assured the husband that hospice was only a phone call away and encouraged him to take one day at a time. The nurse also stated she would phone the husband later that evening to assess how things were going and that she would return that evening if needed.

Because M.B. was actively dying and she was at high risk for increased intensity of her pain, nausea, and dyspnea, a hospice nurse visited M.B. each day to assess her symptoms, the effectiveness of the medication plan, and how the family was coping. Because her husband was unable to administer suppositories, nursing visits were timed so that the nurse could administer one of the daily suppositories, and her sister and mother were able to administer the others.

Three days after her admission to home hospice, M.B. became extremely restless. The nurse assessed that the restlessness might be due to an increase in pain and obtained a physician's order to begin long-acting morphine rectally every 12 hours (to be given in the morning and evening with the antiemetic suppositories). Although the increase in analgesia seemed to relieve the restlessness for awhile, it recurred a day later. No specific cause for this restlessness was identified, but it was considered to represent the delirium seen with terminal agitation. (Terminal agitation is an observable syndrome characterized by inability to rest occurring in clients with varying diagnoses during the last days of life.[1]) M.B. was started on pentobarbital suppositories every 8 hours for her terminal agitation. With careful planning involving the hospice team, the medication schedule for M.B. was maintained despite the fact that six suppositories needed to be administered each day. M.B.'s pain, restlessness, and nausea were controlled until she died peacefully in her home.

REFERENCES

1. March PA. Terminal restlessness. *American Journal of Hospice & Palliative Care.* 1998;15(1):51-53.
2. Given B, Given C. Family home care for individuals with cancer. *Oncology.* 1994; 8(5):77-93.
3. Taylor E, Ferrell B, Grant M, Cheyney L. Managing cancer pain at home: the decisions and ethical conflicts of patients, family caregivers, and homecare nurses. *Oncology Nursing Forum.* 1993;20:919-927.
4. Kazanowski M. Commitment to the end: family caregivers' medication management of symptoms in patients with cancer near death. Doctoral dissertation. Chestnut Hill, Mass: Boston College; 1998.

BIBLIOGRAPHY

Petrin R. The symptom relief kit for hospice patients. *International Journal of Pharmaceutical Compounding.* 1998;Mar/Apr:116-117.

Steele R, Fitch M. Needs of family caregivers of patients receiving home hospice care for cancer. *Oncology Nursing Forum.* 1996;23:823-828.

Case Study Questions

1. What should the nurse do about Mr. B's perceived inability to administer medications?
2. Name two priority symptoms (other than pain and nausea) for which the hospice nurse would assess M.B.
3. How does the nurse instruct family caregivers to assess M.B. for pain?
4. How will the nurse evaluate the effectiveness of the medication management plan?
5. Describe one strategy that home hospice nurses can use to assist family caregivers with medication management of commonly occurring symptoms?

Multiple-Choice Questions

1. Your client, who is actively dying, begins to show signs of restlessness and agitation. Your priority at this time is to assess for:
   A. Fatigue
   B. Hunger
   C. Pain
   D. Terminal agitation

2. In the home, family caregivers assume most of the responsibility for treating a dying person's pain. A factor that would prompt family caregivers to administer a medication for pain would be:
   A. Utilization of rectal route
   B. Fear of overdosing the patient
   C. The client's inability to speak
   D. The perception that the person is suffering

3. What is the purpose of logging the times and amounts of medications given to a client near death:
   A. To evaluate the competency of family caregivers
   B. To identify substance abuse
   C. To assess for potential overdosing of medications
   D. To help in evaluating the effectiveness of symptom management

4. The most frequent symptoms of distress near death are:
   A. Fear, nausea, constipation, and pain
   B. Fear, pain, dyspnea, and fatigue
   C. Pain, dyspnea, delirium, nausea, and vomiting
   D. Pain, constipation, urinary tract spasms

5. Which of the following medications is most appropriate for treatment of terminal agitation:
   A. Hyoscyamine (Levsin)
   B. Morphine sulfate
   C. Pentobarbital
   D. Prochlorperazine

CASE STUDY ANSWERS

1. The nurse must help the husband and mother identify who might be able to administer medications during the time that the mother is not available. The nurse should request medications (and routes) that are most conducive to the caregivers' abilities. For example, family caregivers may express aversion to and perceived difficulty in administering rectal suppositories. Some family caregivers, however, may be open to learning and using this route. Clients may also have an aversion to the rectal route, although the assumption that all clients have this aversion should not be made. Some clients may actually prefer the rectal route, for example if oral medications cause nausea. Intramuscular or subcutaneous injections are generally avoided in clients at the end of life because of the pain they inflict.

2. Shortness of breath is a major symptom of distress at the end of life. M.B. has an increased risk for this because of her diagnosis of lung cancer. Agitation or delirium are other major symptoms of distress near death.

3. Family caregivers should ask the client if she is having pain, where the pain is located, and if possible, have the client rate her pain on a 0 to 10 scale, with 0 indicating no pain and 10 indicating severe pain. If the client is not able to speak about her pain, the nurse instructs the family to watch for objective signs of pain such as grimacing, moaning, or restlessness, and administer medication for pain when any of these symptoms occur.

4. To evaluate the effectiveness of the medication management plan, the nurse asks the family to keep a written log of the times, types, and amounts of each medication administered for each symptom. The nurse visits M.B. as needed, often daily near death, to perform a skilled assessment for pain, dyspnea, and other symptoms indicating discomfort (eg, bladder distention).

5. One strategy to assist family caregivers with management of commonly occurring symptoms would be to develop a set schedule to administer specific medications around the clock, as opposed to PRN. This scheduling of medications eliminates some of the family's decision-making about administering medications.

MULTIPLE-CHOICE ANSWERS

1. C. There are multiple causes of restlessness and agitation near the end of life. Pain is one cause, and it is a priority to assess if it is the cause of the restlessness. The health care provider often administers an analgesic to determine if pain is the cause of the restlessness. Resolution of the agitation supports the premise that pain was the cause.

2. D. Research shows that family caregivers' perception that a symptom indicates suffering will be a facilitating factor to their administering medication. Barriers to treat-

fering will be a facilitating factor to their administering medication. Barriers to treatment include the client's inability to report the symptom and fear of overdosing or harming the client. Some family caregivers have an aversion to using the rectal route to administer medications.

3.   D. Although family caregivers have demonstrated commitment to clients' comfort near death, they do not administer as-needed medications as frequently as they could be given. They should not, however, be evaluated in terms of their competency. Health care providers should recognize that family caregivers can be effective in management of medications despite their uncertainties, fears that they will overmedicate, and their lack of clinical decision-making abilities.

Family caregivers are asked to keep a log or diary of the times, types, and amounts of medication given to evaluate the effectiveness of symptom management.

4.   C. Although fatigue, constipation, and urinary symptoms have been identified as symptoms of distress near death, their incidence is not as high as pain, dyspnea, delirium, nausea, and vomiting. Fear is likely present in many, but it has not often been identified as a "symptom." It is likely related to a symptom such as restlessness or agitation.

5.   C. Hyoscyamine (Levsin) is an anticholinergic used to reduce secretion production. Morphine sulfate is used for pain or dyspnea. Morphine would be appropriate for treatment of agitation if pain were the etiology. The term *terminal agitation* is usually used when a specific cause for agitation cannot be determined.

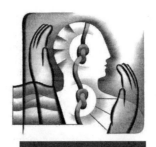

Index